LIBRARY OF VETERINARY PRACTICE

Diseases of
Domestic Guinea Pigs

V.C.G. RICHARDSON MA VetMB MRCVS

OXFORD

BLACKWELL SCIENTIFIC PUBLICATIONS

LONDON EDINBURGH BOSTON

MELBOURNE PARIS BERLIN VIENNA

© 1992 by
Blackwell Scientific Publications
Editorial Offices:
Osney Mead, Oxford OX2 0EL
25 John Street, London WC1N 2BL
23 Ainslie Place, Edinburgh EH3 6AJ
3 Cambridge Center, Cambridge
  Massachusetts 02142, USA
54 University Street, Carlton
  Victoria 3053, Australia

Other Editorial Offices:
Librairie Arnette SA
2, rue Casimir-Delavigne
75006 Paris
France

Blackwell Wissenschafts-Verlag
Meinekestrasse 4
D-1000 Berlin 15
Germany

Blackwell MZV
Feldgasse 13
A-1238 Wien
Austria

First published 1992

Set by Setrite Typesetters, Hong Kong
Printed and bound in Great Britain by
Hartnolls Ltd, Bodmin, Cornwall

DISTRIBUTORS

Marston Book Services Ltd
PO Box 87
Oxford OX2 0DT
(*Orders*: Tel. 0865 791155
       Fax: 0865 791927
       Telex: 837515)

USA
Blackwell Scientific Publications, Inc.
3 Cambridge Center
Cambridge, MA 02142
(*Orders*: Tel: 800 759−6102
         617 225−0401)

Canada
Times Mirror Professional
Publishing, Ltd
5240 Finch Avenue East
Scarborough, Ontario M1S 5A2
(*Orders*: Tel: 800 268−4178
         416 298−1588)

Australia
Blackwell Scientific Publications
(Australia) Pty Ltd
54 University Street
Carlton, Victoria 3053
(*Orders*: Tel: 03 347−0300)

British Library
Cataloguing in Publication Data

Richardson, V.C.G.
  Diseases of domestic guinea pigs. −
  (Library of veterinary practice).
  I. Title II. Series
  599.3234

  ISBN 0−632−03301−0

Contents

Preface, vii

1 The Skin, 1
  1.1 Specific skin conditions, 1

2 The Reproductive System, 15
  2.1 Anatomy, 15
  2.2 Reproductive physiology, 17
  2.3 Pregnancy, 19
  2.4 Infertility, 34

3 The Urinary System, 39
  3.1 Anatomy, 39
  3.2 Physiology, 40
  3.3 Symptoms of urinary tract disorders, 40

4 The Respiratory System, 45
  4.1 Anatomy and physiology, 45
  4.2 Symptoms of respiratory disorders, 45
  4.3 Respiratory infections, 46

5 The Digestive System, 49
  5.1 Anatomy, 49
  5.2 Physiology, 50

6 The Musculoskeletal System, 61

7 The Head and Neck, 68
  7.1 The eye, 68
  7.2 The ear, 72
  7.3 The mouth, 74
  7.4 The neck, 78

8 Behaviour and the Central Nervous System, 81

9   Husbandry, 84
    9.1   Housing, 84
    9.2   Nutrition, 86

10 Anaesthetics and Surgical Preparations, 97
    10.1 Inhalational anaesthetics, 98
    10.2 Injectable anaesthetics, 99

11 Treatments, 103
    11.1   Antibiotics, 105
    11.2   Probiotics, 108
    11.3   Fluid therapy, 109
    11.4   Anti-fungal agents, 109
    11.5   Anti-diarrhoeal preparations, 110
    11.6   Topical preparations, 111
    11.7   Eye preparations, 112
    11.8   Ectoparasitic preparations, 113
    11.9   Endoparasitic preparations, 115
    11.10 Miscellaneous treatments, 116
    11.11 Vitamin preparations, 118
    11.12 Cleansing solutions, 119

12 Zoonotic Aspects, 121

    Appendix: Miscellaneous Physiological Data, 123

    Further Reading, 125

    Index, 126

Preface

I have bred and exhibited guinea pigs for over 20 years, and since I qualified as a veterinary surgeon I have been able to expand this interest in a more professional capacity. This book aims to provide a comprehensive text covering all aspects of the species, and it is written in part to try and help dispel the myth that 'a sick guinea pig is a dead guinea pig'. It is hoped that it will be of help to veterinary surgeons in general practice, and also to anyone who shares an interest in guinea pigs.

The scientific name of the guinea pig is *Cavia porcellus*, from which their other name, the cavy, originates. When I was reviewing the references in preparation for this book 'guinea pig' emerged as the most popular term and that is why I have chosen to use it throughout my text.

I have tried to make the information as readily accessible as possible, and wherever a treatment is mentioned it is given a reference number in brackets. All these treatments are listed numerically in Chapter 11 which provides full details of dose rates, contraindications, etc., and also the components of the proprietary preparations which should enable like alternatives to be found, if the former are unavailable.

There are many people who I would like to thank: those who have given me advice on some of the treatments mentioned, my many friends and fellow exhibitors, and especially my colleague and husband Ean, for his patience, encouragement and help in preparing the manuscript. I am also grateful to Wayne Chant for providing the illustrations.

V.C.G.R.

1/ The Skin

The skin of the guinea pig normally provides a resistant barrier against infection. However, there are many factors which lower this resistance and predispose the guinea pig to the development of skin disease. One of the most common findings is an increased incidence of skin problems in guinea pigs fed on marginal diets, especially if these diets have a low vitamin C content. The feeding of stale dried food will cause such a problem as the vitamin C content deteriorates rapidly 6–9 weeks after milling. Rabbit food is also too low in vitamin C to be used as a staple diet for cavies.

Other important stresses, which predispose the guinea pig to the development of skin conditions, are overheating, pregnancy and showing.

1.1 Specific skin conditions

Ringworm

Clinical signs. Areas of alopecia, usually accompanied by varying degrees of seborrhoea. The lesions are often found around the face but may spread to the rest of the body. The affected hair can be readily plucked from its follicles. The condition may or may not be puritic. There may also be accompanying lesions on the owner.

Diagnosis. The causal agent is usually *Tricophyton mentagrophytes* or *Microsporum gypseum* so it will not fluoresce under ultraviolet light (Wood's lamp). Direct microscopic examination of hair from the lesion together with culture on Sabouraud's medium will confirm the diagnosis.

Treatment. Griseofulvin (Tx 18) at a dose of 25 mg/kg (approximately 0.75 mg/kg of feed) for 4–6 weeks is generally effective. If griseofulvin is used to treat an individual animal it is best given orally on a daily basis, and the approximate dose is an eighth of a teaspoon daily, which can be given mixed with an unsaturated fatty acid supplement (e.g. 0.5 ml Norderm, Norden Laboratories). Care must be taken when using griseofulvin in very young animals (under 3 months) as a high incidence of infant mortality has been reported in association with the use of this anti-fungal preparation in one colony. Griseofulvin should also not be administered to pregnant sows.

Alternatively tolnaftate 1% (Tx 19, Tinaderm-M cream) can be applied to the lesions twice daily until they resolve.

Cases with severe accompanying seborrhoea will benefit from the use of an anti-fungal shampoo, e.g. hexetidine 0.5% (Tx 47). This shampoo is most effective if it is left in contact with the skin for some time (1−2 hours in severely affected cases) before rinsing.

A diet with good vitamin C content must be fed at the same time as treating with any anti-fungal agent to enable the affected guinea pig to make a full recovery.

Other mycoses

Clinical signs. Guinea pigs may suffer from a range of other mycotic infections, and the clinical signs may vary from mild skin changes indistinguishable from mange in its early stages, to very severe seborrhoea with accompanying systemic signs including cystitis, pneumonia, convulsions and reproductive disorders.

Diagnosis. Microscopic examination of the hair and culture on Sabouraud's medium.

Cases which are suggestive of mycotic infection are those which do not respond to the standard anti-parasitic treatment.

Treatment. Griseofulvin (as for ringworm) and the use of an anti-fungal shampoo, e.g. 0.5% hexetidine (Tx 47). The shampoo should be left in contact with the skin for as long as possible (up to 2 hours) before rinsing. The effectiveness of the treatment will be increased if all the affected hairs are plucked from the guinea pig's body as this will remove a high percentage of the fungal spores. This treatment can be repeated every 3−4 days as necessary.

The use of amphotericin B has been reported in those cases exhibiting severe systemic involvement.

Mange

This condition may also be called 'sellnick' or 'rat mange'. It refers to the condition produced by *Trixacarus caviae*, a sarcoptiform mite.

Clinical signs. These usually occur 3−5 weeks after infection, although it may remain inapparent for considerable periods. The lesions are seen mainly around the head and shoulders and over the dorsum but may spread further to affect the whole guinea pig. The hair comes out and the skin is seborrhoeic and usually intensely pruritic. There may also be many open sores due to self-trauma. If the sow is in-pig and is quite severely affected she may resorb or abort her litter. If her young are born normally they will become infected immediately.

In cases where the pruritus is severe the guinea pig may also exhibit nervous signs, and in extreme cases may actually have fits.

Diagnosis. Microscopic examination of skin scrapings.

Treatment. Numerous treatments have been advocated. Probably the most effective is ivermectin (Tx 36), but as this is not licensed for guinea pigs it should be used with care. The dose is 200 µg/kg and this can be repeated at 10−14-day intervals if necessary. The Ivomec injection for cattle (Merck, Sharp & Dohme Ltd (MSD)) is the most convenient preparation to use (0.02 ml/kg) and it can be diluted 1 : 10 to produce a dose of 0.2 ml which should be administered subcutaneously. Alternatively this same drug has been administered orally with the same effect. Up to 2 drops from a 2 ml syringe (equivalent to 400 µg) can be given with no side-effects. Although the oral absorption of ivermectin has not been evaluated treatment in this way seems to be effective.

Trials using ivermectin, performed at the Cambridge Cavy Trust have shown that greater doses of this drug can be used without any adverse effects. Their recommendations are as follows:
- Age 3 weeks to 3 months: 0.1 ml (1000 µg) by subcutaneous injection. Oral dosing not recommended.
- Age 3 months to adult: 0.2 ml by subcutaneous injection. One drop given orally.

These treatments can be repeated after an interval of 10−14 days.

Other preparations which can be used include sprays containing pyrethrum extract (e.g. Johnson's Anti-Pest Insect spray).

Quellada (Tx 38, gamma benzene hexachloride 1%) shampoo has been advocated for use weekly. This must be thoroughly rinsed off the coat. Seleen (Tx 35) can also be used as a shampoo.

Tetmosol solution (Tx 37), a human scabies preparation available from chemists, is also very effective. It must be diluted 1 : 72 (approximately one tablespoon of Tetmosol to a litre of water) and the whole guinea pig should be dipped in this solution. It should not be rinsed off but allowed to dry on the coat. This treatment can be repeated fortnightly. Tetmosol is also available as a soap but this is less effective as it must be washed off thoroughly. Tetmosol at the dilution recommended above can also be used to clean out the living quarters of the affected guinea pig.

If this or any other skin condition is accompanied by intense pruritus, this can be controlled by an injection of a steroid preparation (Tx 44 and 45). Creams containing local anaesthetic agents can also be used on the lesions to prevent self-trauma.

Self-trauma can also be limited if the hindfeet are lightly dressed, or alternatively the worst sores can be protected with a loose body bandage.

If nervous signs are present Diazepam (Tx 51) at a dose of 1–2 mg/kg can be given intramuscularly to help control these. However, if the symptoms are as severe as this, euthanasia may have to be considered.

An alternative treatment for controlling any seizures is primidone (Mysoline Tx 49).

If a pregnant sow is badly affected she should be treated. The slight risks incurred by handling a gravid sow are better than the consequences of leaving her untreated. Ivermectin has been administered during pregnancy without obvious side effects, and dosing is a less stressful procedure than bathing or dipping.

If the problem is a recurrent one, treatment is more effective if it is varied. If the same preparation is used repeatedly it is not unknown for some mites to develop resistance to the treatment and the condition then becomes more persistent.

Comment. Trixacarus caviae is a burrowing mite and transmission can be via direct or indirect contact. The female burrows into the skin and lays her eggs in the tunnels she creates. Multiple larvae then hatch out in these tunnels, metamorphose through two nymph stages and then develop into adults. The life cycle takes 14 days. Stresses such as malnutrition, overcrowding, poor ventilation, extreme heat and pregnancy predispose to this condition.

Prevention. If there is a problem in the caviary all individuals can be treated with ivermectin (Tx 36) given orally in order to eradicate any sub-clinical disease.

Demodex

Clinical signs. Areas of alopecia, especially around the head and forelegs. The condition may or may not be pruritic.

Diagnosis. Microscopic examination of skin scrapings.

Treatment. Injection of a high dose of ivermectin (Tx 36) which may need to be repeated 2−3 times at fortnightly intervals.

Lice

Clinical signs. This condition need not be pruritic, and the lice can often be seen in the fur. 'Static lice' refers to the eggs of the lice which are seen as black or white specks sticking to the hair, especially around the neck and ears and on the ventral abdomen. 'Running lice' refers to the adult forms which are visible to the naked eye.

In some cases the term static lice is used to describe the fur mite *Chirodiscoides caviae* (see below).

Diagnosis. Microscopic examination of hair and skin scrapings.

Treatment. Quellada (Tx 38) or a spray containing pyrethrum extract (e.g. Johnson's Anti-Pest Insect spray). Seleen (Tx 35) will also be effective. Both Quellada and Seleen can be repeated at weekly intervals. A more old-fashioned remedy was to use oil of sassafras, but unfortunately this oil is no longer readily obtainable. It can be worked gently into the coat avoiding the eyes and genitals and left to evaporate. It will kill the lice and their eggs and leave the coat in a glossy condition. The treatment can be repeated after 14 days.

Comment. Causal agents are varied. Infestations with *Gyropus ovalis*, *Trimenopen jenningsi* and *Gliricola porcelli* have been recorded.

Gliricola porcelli is the most common. The adults are yellow−grey in colour and are up to 1.5 mm long. *Gyropus ovalis* are similar, but are slightly smaller and they have a less rounded head. *Trimenopen jenningsi* is thought to be of little pathogenic significance unless the guinea pig is stressed.

Fur mite

These mites (*Chirodiscoides caviae*) are 0.5 mm long and are often found joined in pairs. They appear to produce no clinical signs even when the guinea pig is heavily infested. They will be removed with any of the ectoparasitic treatments recommended above for mange and lice.

Prevention. The load of ectoparasites can be reduced by hanging a Vapona sticky strip (containing dichlorvos) in the environment for a 48-hour period once a week. Nuvan Top, a spray containing dichlorvos for use in cats and dogs *should not* be used on guinea pigs. The active ingredients are powerful cholinesterase inhibitors and toxicity is likely to develop. If Nuvan Top has been used the antidote is atropine sulphate which should be administered at a dose of 0.1 mg/kg given intraperitoneally

'Broken back'

Clinical signs. A single area of hair loss in the centre of the back which may become an open sore, if left will scab over. This condition is often mistakenly assumed to be mange. It seems to be associated with stresses such as showing or pregnancy.

Treatment. Bathe the sore with a dilute saline solution (Tx 59) and dry. Dermisol cream or Vetsovate (Tx 25 or 28) can be applied topically up to three times daily. However, the condition will resolve with bathing only. Once the lesion is healed the affected skin may be fairly dry and this can be conditioned by topical application of cod-liver oil or evening primrose oil.

Comment. This condition affects lighter coloured guinea pigs most frequently and it is thought to occur as a result of the guinea pig 'overheating'. Barley is a particularly 'overheating food', as is flaked maize and these should be removed from the diet. An excess of rabbit pellets has also been implicated as a cause of overheating. The problem is seen at its worst in the heat of the summer.

'Post-natal sores'

This condition is similar to 'broken back' and develops in some sows after parturition as a sore in the centre of the back and it can be treated in the same manner. It is thought to be due to a mineral and protein deficiency.

In late pregnancy sows prone to developing this condition can be given some Bemax as a supplement sprinkled on their food. Alternatively they can be given a bread and milk mash to which extra soya flour has been added to provide supplementary protein. A couple of drops of Vitapet daily as a source of polyunsaturated oils may also be beneficial. This condition will also respond if 1−2 drops of Abidec (Tx 52), a vitamin preparation, are given orally once a day.

Comment. This condition also occurs in sows during gestation and is also likely to be due to a mineral and protein deficiency. The treatment is the same as for 'broken back'.

Skin lesions immediately after parturition

Clinical signs. Sows develop raw patches on their rumps and ventral abdomen soon after parturition.

Comment. This condition is more prevalent if the sow has had a long and difficult labour. She becomes caked in blood and uterine fluids because she is too tired to clean herself immediately after the birth. This then begins to irritate her and she tears the hair out from the affected area; the lesions are therefore due to self-trauma.

There is also a possible inherited tendency towards developing this condition.

Treatment. It is important to check the sow after the birth and if necessary clean her with a dilute solution of Savlon (Tx 58).

If raw patches do develop they must be cleaned gently and towelled dry. Antibiotic creams should be used with extreme caution as there is a real risk that they will be ingested by the youngsters whilst suckling and therefore these preparations are probably best avoided. If the sores are weeping, calamine lotion can be applied and this should dry up the lesions in 24 hours with less risk to the youngsters. Some sources suggest the application of cod-liver oil to the bald areas to help them heal, but this should be avoided due to the risk of vitamin D overdose if ingested by the suckling youngsters.

Seborrhoea

Seborrhoea and the presence of excess scurf in the coat may be a symptom of many different conditions, notably mange, ringworm and other mycotic infections, and chronic liver disorders. The presence of this scurf is in itself intensely pruritic irrespective of the causal agent.

Treatment. As well as treating the underlying cause, the scurf can be removed by using a tar-based shampoo, e.g. Tarlite (Tx 50). Shampooing can be repeated at weekly intervals and the resultant improvement will bring great relief to the affected guinea pig.

If it is difficult to determine whether the initiating cause is parasitic or fungal in origin it is advisable to use Quellada (Tx 38) and Hexocil (Tx 47) as a combined wash, or alternatively Seleen (Tx 35) which has both antiparasitic and antifungal properties.

Alopecia

During pregnancy

Some sows lose their hair during pregnancy. The symptoms begin in middle to late pregnancy and the hair just begins to fall out. There is no accompanying pruritus. If a sow has experienced this condition once she is likely to do so during subsequent pregnancies and the condition is also worse in older and frequently bred females.

Treatment. Vitamin B supplementation has been advocated, either in the form of a weekly multivitamin injection or as daily drops of an oral preparation. However, the condition will resolve slowly after parturition without treatment.

Post-natal

After parturition some sows may lose most of their coat. The hair is lost bilaterally from the flanks and ventral abdomen.

Occasionally the young may actually be responsible for pulling hair from their dams.

Treatment. None is required. This condition is thought to be hormonal in origin and will correct itself once the sow stops nursing her litter.

Liver disease

Clinical signs. The hair cover is sparse and the skin may be thickened. There is often accompanying seborrhoea. Pruritus is not usually a feature unless the seborrhoea is severe. The guinea pig may twitch frequently.

Severe, untreated mycosis will also present with similar clinical signs.

Treatment. If parasitic and fungal causes are eliminated then this condition is often a sign of underlying liver disease. If the seborrhoea is intense a tar and sulphur based shampoo (Tarlite Tx 50) is very effective and this can be repeated weekly as necessary. Other treatment is supportive and should include a vitamin and unsaturated fatty acid supplement, e.g. Vitapet. However, in severe cases exhibiting nervous signs the prognosis is poor.

Scurvy

One of the manifestations of this condition is hair loss, usually accompanied with the other symptoms of weight loss, lameness, weakness and bleeding from the gums.

Treatment. Vitamin C at a dose of 100 mg/kg preferably given orally in drop form until the condition resolves.

Comment. In any skin condition the provision of adequate vitamin C is of paramount importance. Plenty of this vitamin is to be found in fresh greens, carrots and beetroot. Rosehip syrup is another useful source of vitamin C. (For further details about this vitamin refer to Chapter 9.)

Hair loss at weaning

Young guinea pigs may get a thin hair coat at weaning time as they lose their neonatal haircoat and it is gradually replaced by mature hair. No treatment is required other than the provision of an adequate diet as this is a completely natural phenomenon.

Chewing

Clinical signs. Hair loss in any area of the body, and the hair is often bitten to the roots. It may be self-inflicted in which case only the areas the guinea pig can reach are affected, or it may be more widespread if the chewing is from other guinea pigs. Guinea pigs that share accommodation with rabbits are often chewed by the rabbit. In one case of a guinea pig kept in an outside run the hair was seen being removed by a robin to provide nesting material!

Treatment. If the condition is self-inflicted it is often a result of boredom and alteration of the guinea pig's environment may break the habit. As, by its nature, the guinea pig is always eating, the provision of ample amounts of good hay will help prevent boredom and stop the development of this vice. If the chewing is being done by other guinea pigs the affected individual should be penned separately. If the hair loss is found in youngsters as a result of overgrooming by their mother the affected young should be weaned as soon as possible.

In some cases of coat chewing in the long-haired breeds (Peruvians, Coronets and Shelties) a vitamin and mineral deficiency has been implicated and these cases have been resolved once 'Stress', a supplement for dogs and cats, has been added to the daily diet.

Urine-scalding

Clinical signs. A moist dermatitis around the genitals ventrally in the female and around the rump in the male. It may be a consequence of polyuria.

Treatment. Twice-daily applications of a combined antibiotic–steroid preparation such as Vetsovate cream (Tx 28) is effective. The affected area can be protected by use of a resistant barrier cream such as zinc and castor oil, or Vaseline.

Epidermoid cyst (sebaceous cyst)

Clinical signs. These cysts can arise anywhere on the body, but are usually found on the back. They are slightly soft when squeezed and if ruptured they discharge their caseous contents.

Treatment. If the cyst ruptures it can be squeezed out and then bathed with a mild saline solution (Tx 59). No extra treatment is needed. If the cysts are irritating the guinea pig then their removal should be considered, although they may recur subsequently. Otherwise they can be left.

Comment. These cysts are derived from hair follicles (not sebaceous glands) and possess a keratinizing epidermal lining which generates the caseous contents.

Abscesses

These may occur anywhere on the body and are often the result of fighting. They must be differentiated from cervical lymphadenitis (see Chapter 7) and pseudotuberculosis. Occasionally a pea-sized lump is felt in the throat which is due to a swollen lymph node and this will regress with time.

A wide range of bacteria have been isolated from such abscesses including *Pseudomonas aeruginosa*, *Pasturella multocida*, *Corynebacterium pyogenes*, *Staphylococcus aureus*, *Streptococcus* spp. and other environmental contaminants (*Enterobacteriaceae*).

Clinical signs. A localized soft swelling originating from a cut or scratch. It may be hot and painful to the touch. They commonly occur in the throat region where they are usually the result of a thistle from the hay penetrating through the mucous membranes of the mouth and tracking under the chin.

Treatment. If the abscess has burst it must be thoroughly bathed with a dilute saline solution (Tx 59), and flushed with a 3% solution of hydrogen peroxide (Tx 56). It is then best to use anti-bacterials topically only, either a cream e.g. Dermisol (Tx 25), or perhaps more conveniently an intramammary preparation to instil antibiotics into the abscess site. The latter has the advantage of a long nozzle to get the antibiotics under the skin even when the wound has closed to a hole of small diameter. If care is taken to use only a small amount of an intramammary preparation (considering its high antibiotic concentration) the response to treatment will be good.

If the abscess has not burst it can be brought to a head with warm poulticing, or by smearing warm magnesium sulphate paste onto the surface of the abscess.

The affected guinea pig must be isolated to prevent other guinea pigs licking the abscess and ingesting the infected material.

Comment. Two adult boars should never be penned together as they will usually fight. However, an older boar may tolerate a younger one if there are no females around and two sibling males may tolerate each other if kept together from birth, but again only if they are alone. It is therefore better to keep a pair of females as females will nearly always live together in harmony.

As abscesses may also arise from scratches caused by sharp flooring or wire doors, or even sharp foodstuffs, e.g. straw. It is important to eliminate these from the hutch to prevent the problem from recurring.

Boils

Clinical signs. These may occur anywhere on the body and appear as subcutaneous fluid-filled swellings. Agoutis seem to be particularly prone to developing this condition.

Treatment. None is necessary, the fluid may resorb or burst on its own. The temptation to drain them should be resisted as there is a likelihood of introducing infection.

Grease gland (scent gland)

This is a wrinkled piece of skin at the base of the spine which is not normally noticeable as it is covered with hair. It sometimes becomes very thick and glutinous due to the grease it secretes. It is much more noticeable in boars than sows and it can become quite dirty. However, it is perfectly normal and is best left alone.

If necessary the thick grease can be removed with surgical spirit or a gel hand cleanser (e.g. Swarfega).

Anal fold dermatitis

Clinical signs. A moist dermatitis in the circumanal skin folds, caused by a build up of secretions of sebum in these folds and subsequent secondary infection.

Treatment. The area should be cleaned with an anti-bacterial agent and then a topical anti-bacterial cream, e.g. Panalog (Tx 27) or Dermisol (Tx 25) can be applied 2−3 times daily until the condition resolves.

Basal cell tumour

Clinical signs. A slow growing mass, which is roughly oval, well-circumscribed, firmly attached to the epidermis, but freely mobile over the underlying tissues. As the mass increases in size it may ulcerate through the skin discharging some of its caeseous contents, and at this time it may become secondarily infected. They can be found anywhere on the body, but are usually seen in the skin of the dorsum or flanks.

Treatment. Surgical excision of the mass will result in a complete cure. If the tumour is entirely resected local recurrence and metastases are rare.

Pathology. Basal cell tumours contain variable degrees of differentiation, and they can differentiate into both squamous epithelium and sebaceous cells. Some cells in the centre may form hair follicle-like structures with a clearly defined zone of mature keratin and these tumours are termed tricofolliculomas.

Comment. These skin tumours are seen fairly frequently and there may be a familial tendency to their development. They are benign tumours, but it is advisable to remove them before they ulcerate.

Fly strike (blowfly myiasis)

Clinical signs. The presence of larvae (maggots) of blowfly colonizing a moist wound. Maggots may also be found under the adjacent skin.

Treatment. Thorough cleansing of the area (Tx 56–57) and removal of all the maggots. Subsequently the wound must be kept clean and dry and an anti-bacterial cream can be applied (Tx 25).

Comment. This condition is relatively uncommon in guinea pigs. However, if the wound is cleaned aggressively and all the maggots removed the prognosis for recovery is good. Guinea pigs, unlike rabbits, seem far less susceptible to the development of the toxic shock associated with the larval secretions.

2/ The Reproductive System

2.1 Anatomy

Figures 2.1 and 2.2 describe the internal anatomy of the reproductive tract of both sexes. An important consideration is that in males the inguinal canals which contain the testes are open throughout the

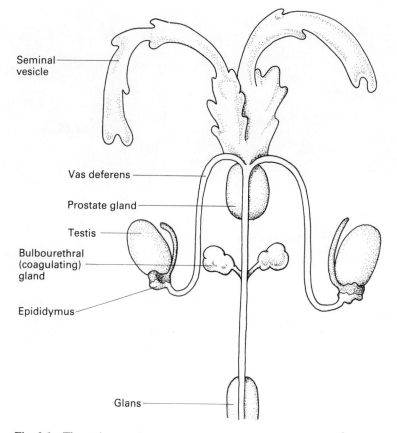

Fig. 2.1 The male reproductive tract.

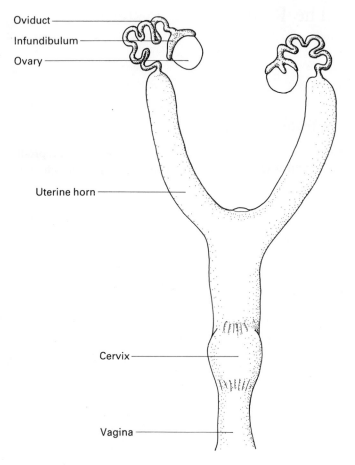

Fig. 2.2 The female reproductive tract.

guinea pig's life, and therefore there is an increased tendency for prolapse of the abdominal organs after castration. In the adult male, the coiled tubular vesicular glands lie ventral to the urethra and extend to a length of approximately 10 cm into the abdominal cavity from their base in the pubic area. They should not be confused with the uterine horns of the female.

There are two mammary glands and the nipples, situated in the groin, are present in both sexes. For details of the external genitalia see opposite.

Sexing

This can be done at any age. The guinea pig is turned onto its back and its weight should be supported with the palm of one hand so that the genitalia can be examined. In both sexes the anus is closely associated to the genitalia. Gentle pressure on either side of the male's sex organs will extrude the penis, whereas in front of the anus in the sow there is a hairless area of skin shaped like an upside-down 'Y' covering the vagina. In front of the vagina is the urethral opening. The vagina is normally closed by a membrane (the hymen) except during oestrus and at parturition.

When the male's penis is extruded there should be two prongs of even length at the end. If these are absent or of unequal length the boar is likely to be sterile.

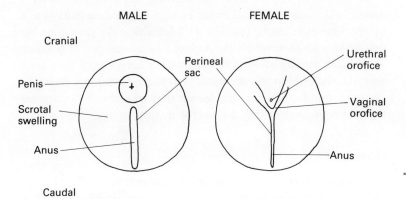

Fig. 2.3 External genitalia.

2.2 Reproductive physiology

Reproductive parameters of the cavy

- Sexual maturity (female): 4−6 weeks.
- Sexual maturity (male): 3−5 weeks.
- Female breeding age: 4−5 months, weight 500 g.
- Male breeding age: 3−5 months, weight 550 g.
- Oestrus cycle: 15−17 days.
- Gestation range: 59−72 days (depending upon litter size).

- Litter size: 1–6 (average 3).
- Birthweight: 100 g each.
- Breeding life of female: 4–5 years.
- Breeding life of male: 5 years or longer.
- Weaning age: 3 weeks.

Breeding

A female can be put with a male once she weighs 500 g, or is 4–5 months old. However she should have her first litter before she reaches 10 months of age because soon after this time her pelvic bones fuse, and her chances of developing dystocia are greatly increased.

Although males are capable of breeding from 4 weeks of age it is advisable not to use them for breeding until they are over 4 months old. Guinea pigs can either be kept as breeding pairs or as a harem. One male can be run with 4–5 females at the same time but two males should never be put together in a large pen of females.

If males are not allowed to mate with a female until they are a year old, their libido will decrease, even to the extent that they may become infertile, and for this reason it is advisable that they are bred from as soon as they are over 4 months of age.

Oestrus

Guinea pigs are polyoestrus, coming into season every 15–17 days, and at this time they exhibit several characteristic changes in their behaviour patterns. The sow may mount other females in the pen and give a purring or mating call as she does this. If she is stroked along the back and rump at this time she will dip her back and purr (the lordosis posture).

Oestrus itself lasts for 24–48 hours and the sow will accept the boar for approximately 6–11 hours during this time. Spontaneous ovulation usually occurs 10 hours after the onset of oestrus. As the sow comes into season her external genitalia swell, and the hymen usually opens the day before oestrus to allow for copulation with the boar. Once the mating has been completed the vagina is sealed by a plug of ejaculate known as the stopper, and this generally remains in place for 48 hours after which time it drops out and the hymen reseals until parturition.

Post-partum oestrus

Sows return to oestrus 6−48 hours after parturition so it is wise to separate the sow and the boar once the sow is pregnant to avoid her being mated again at this time. Carrying a second litter whilst rearing the first would be harmful. (80% of matings at this time are fertile.)

2.3 Pregnancy

Gestation ranges from 59−72 days depending upon the size of the litter. If the litter is large the gestation is likely to be shorter, whereas conversely smaller litters are carried for a longer time.

The size of the litter is determined by the sow, and there is an inherited tendency to produce either large or small litters. The optimum litter size is three. Very small litters (one to two young) carry an increased chance of dystocia due to fetal oversize, whereas large litters lead to the birth of small and often weakly youngsters.

Pregnancy diagnosis

Pregnancy can be determined by monitoring the sow's weight as there is usually a considerable increase during gestation, often up to twice her normal weight. However handling, and therefore weighing, of the pregnant sow must be kept to the minimum to avoid any possible complications during her pregnancy. By careful abdominal palpation the first fetal movements can be felt at 42 days (these first movements are termed 'quickening') and at 50 days very definite movements can be felt. These continue throughout gestation until the last week when the uterus has become so gravid that the movement of the fetuses becomes restricted and in some cases may not be felt at all.

This examination must be undertaken very gently, the sow being held around the shoulders with one hand whilst her abdomen rests on the palm of the other hand. No digital pressure is necessary, the movements will be felt if the palm is cupped around the sow's body.

From 6 weeks of gestation fetal skeletons are visible radiographically, but radiography should not be necessary to detect pregnancy and may be harmful if inadvertently done before this date. However radiography can be useful to check sows that are overdue (those that have been over 70 days without a boar) as in some cases a sow may resorb all or part of a litter but still continue to look pregnant.

Superfetation

This phenomenon has been recorded in guinea pigs. It is possible for the sow to carry fetuses from two separate fertilization events occurring at different oestruses. In most cases a second fertile mating occurs at the subsequent oestrus, however in several cases sows have produced two litters 35 days apart, (the second litter being produced from fertilized ova shed two oestrus cycles later). The uterus has two separate horns and each litter is carried in a different horn. It is quite possible for both litters to be reared successfully.

Pseudopregnancy

This condition is rare but has been recorded in guinea pigs. Its duration is approximately 17 days.

Sows which miscarry their litters early in gestation may continue to look pregnant and may actually begin to produce milk. Despite the absence of young such sows may produce milk for 1−2 weeks and great care must be taken to ensure that they do not develop mastitis during this time. If the sow is not fed any greens her milk flow will soon decrease and it is advisable to withhold all such green food until the condition resolves.

Special nutritional considerations of the pregnant sow

1 During her pregnancy the sow's requirements for vitamin C increases twofold from 10 mg/kg/day to 20 mg/kg/day. This can be supplied by adding soluble vitamin C tablets (e.g. Redoxon Tx 54) to the drinking water (the average guinea pig drinks 85 ml/day). Alternatively rosehip syrup or blackcurrant juice can be added to the water bottles. However most commercial pellets will provide adequate vitamin C provided that they have not been stored for a prolonged period (greater than 3 months). Beetroot and carrots contain 3 mg per 25 g of vitamin C, and most cabbages, broccoli and spinach 17 mg per 25 g of vitamin C, so supplementation may

only be necessary in the winter when green food is scarce. Youngsters born to vitamin C deficient mothers may have paralysed hindquarters and swollen painful joints.

2   It is important that the sow does not become obese as this will predispose her to developing pregnancy toxaemia. She must be allowed access to plenty of good hay and grass which will be filling but of less calorific value than concentrates. Eating large quantities of molasses-enriched food will similarly lead to obesity, as will flaked maize which is very calorific. She must not be kept in cramped surroundings but encouraged to exercise.

3   Raspberry leaves are often fed by breeders during gestation and are said to ensure ease of parturition. Various raspberry products are certainly used for this reason in other species and the author feels that they are a useful supplement during pregnancy. They also have mild astringent properties.

4   Bran fed in the form of a mash is a useful component of the diet but care must be taken not to overfeed this cereal as it is high in phosphorus and low in calcium and will lead to the development of weak young with undermineralized skeletons.

Complications during pregnancy

Pregnancy toxaemia

Clinical signs. The sow stops eating, becomes depressed, and adopts a hunched, ruffled appearance. She may salivate profusely and the characteristic smell of ketones can be detected on her breath as she becomes ketoacidotic. The condition progresses to muscle spasms and death. The symptoms often occur abruptly, and the condition is more prevalent in hot weather.

Pathology. Laboratory findings include aciduria, proteinuria and hyperlipaemia. Microscopically there is a fatty degeneration of the liver and at post-mortem this organ looks pale yellow and is enlarged and very friable. The blood is lactescent (fatty) and the adrenal glands may be enlarged and haemorrhagic.

Treatment. Treatment is rarely successful in advanced cases. In the early stages administration of a glucose or propylene glycol solution may prove beneficial (e.g. Ketol). In later stages an injection of steroids such as betamethasone or dexamethasone (Tx 44 and 45) and administration of up to 10 ml fluids subcutaneously (4% or 5% glucose—saline Tx 15) can be attempted. An intramuscular injection of vitamin B_{12} (Tx 55) may act as an effective appetite stimulant.

Comment. Pregnancy toxaemia is a metabolic disorder similar to that observed in sheep prior to parturition (twin lamb disease). Predisposing factors are obesity and any stress which may induce temporary anorexia in late pregnancy. The sow goes into negative energy balance. She is unable to supply sufficient glucose to the developing fetuses from the products of digestion and begins to catabolize her own tissues. This progresses to the development of ketoacidosis. It is therefore very important to keep stresses such as handling and weighing to the absolute mininum.

There is evidence to suggest that sub-clinical hypocalcaemia may predispose to the development of ketosis and calcium supplementation during the last week of pregnancy and first week of lactation will reduce the incidence of this disease.

Ketosis is also seen in obese animals and older males after stress. The treatment is the same as for the pregnant sow.

Prevention. The sow must be housed in a hutch large enough to provide room for exercise and must not be allowed to become obese. In-pig sows can be given water in which a little glucose has been dissolved as a ready supply of this sugar in late pregnancy. An alternative preventative measure is to add a small amount of liquid Lectade to the drinking water of pregnant sows (this product is also used to treat twin lamb disease in sheep). The required dilution of this is 20 ml of Lectade into 250 ml of water (Tx 16).

Calcium supplementation (Tx 53) can be given orally during the last week of pregnancy and the first week of lactation.

Resorption

Clinical signs. This may occur before pregnancy has been detected and therefore go unnoticed, it just being assumed that the sow is taking her time in conceiving, or that she is infertile. Any stress such as a sudden diet change may lead to resorption, as will a period of poor feeding. Sows with severe mange mite infestation are quite likely either to resorb or abort their litters. If fetal loss occurs in the very early stages of gestation the sow may not outwardly appear sick.

Treatment. Avoidance of sudden stress and provision of an adequate diet should prevent the occurrence of resorption.

Miscarriage and abortion

Clinical signs. This occurs when the fetuses have reached a later stage in their development. If it occurs fairly early in gestation (up to around 40 days) the sow need not be systemically affected and all that may be noticed is that she has traces of blood around her face acquired from cleaning herself. Later in gestation she is more likely to become noticeably ill; there may be severe blood loss at the same time, and this may prove fatal. It is however possible at any stage of gestation that only part of the litter is lost, and if the sow's condition improves it is possible that she can carry the rest of the litter to term and give birth normally.

Treatment. This may be unsuccessful if the sow is seriously ill. She must be placed in isolation. Supportive therapy, warmth and good food are necessary to maintain the pregnancy if only part of the litter is lost. An injection of vitamin B_{12} (Tx 55) may prove beneficial.

If there are any dead fetuses or placentas left inside the uterus, an injection of $1-2$ iu oxytocin (Tx 48) can be given intramuscularly to aid their expulsion.

Comment. If a sow has had an abortion or miscarriage she must be rested and allowed to regain her strength for at least 2 months before being allowed to breed again. However, if the sow is in good condition despite having lost a litter at term she can either be used as a foster mother or put back with a boar to prevent her moping or becoming distressed whilst searching for her babies.

Abortions and premature births can also occur if the pregnant sow is penned with other nursing sows. As the pregnant sow takes interest in and cleans the other youngsters she may start having early contractions resulting in the loss of her litter. Parturition can be induced in this way from as early as the 5th week of gestation. It is therefore advisable to separate pregnant sows to prevent this problem.

High environmental temperatures have also been linked to an increased incidence of abortion. Sows that are exposed to a temperature of over 32°C (90°F) for an hour a day are at risk of losing their litters. It is very important to keep the caviary cool, especially during the hot summer months when most of the breeding takes place.

Abortion and resorption can occur as a consequence of a systemic infection and have been associated with *Bordetella bronchiseptica*, *Streptococcus pneumoniae* and *Salmonella* infections.

Premature births

Clinical signs. The young are born small and weak, with short and very silky soft hair and their nails are usually white. The sow will probably be unwell. Any birth which occurs before day 60 of gestation is premature. It occurs if the sow is in poor condition or is subject to a sudden stress. Premature births are also more common in sows that have been bred too young, i.e. sows under 5 months old.

Treatment. As long as the sow is not too weak she can be brought back to health with careful nursing and good feeding.

Intra-uterine haemorrhage

Clinical signs. The pregnant sow rapidly becomes unthrifty and she has a bloody discharge from the vulva.

Pathology. One or both horns of the gravid uterus will be full of blood, and the fetuses will be dead.

Comment. The aetiology of this condition is unknown, although it may be the result of a disorder of liver metabolism. Streptococcal infection has also been implicated.

Prevention. The animal must not be allowed to become obese as this will compromise liver function.

The hormonal maintenance of pregnancy

The successful initiation of pregnancy depends upon an extended secretion of luteal progesterone. The absolute requirement for progesterone persists throughout gestation and a balance of both this hormone and oestrogen are necessary to maintain the pregnancy to full term. In many species these steroid hormones are provided by the ovarian corpus luteum, which is under higher control from the maternal pituitary, and removal of the ovaries or the pituitary leads to abortion. In the guinea pig however, the pregnancy does not depend totally upon ovarian–pituitary interactions and these organs can be removed during the pregnancy without causing abortion. Experiments have shown that the pituitary is important for the first 3 days, and the ovaries for the first 28 days. Thereafter the majority of oestrogen and progesterone is synthesized in the placenta.

Comment. Stress and malnutrition in the first month will result in decreased activity of the ovaries, and it may be the result of insufficient hormone secretion by these under-functioning gonads that leads to early resorption.

Parturition

Parturition usually occurs 18–20 days after the first definite movements are felt. However, the actual onset of parturition is often difficult to predict, although there is sometimes evidence of nesting behaviour by the sow. There may also be subtle mood changes probably associated with the pains of first stage labour. Prior to parturition the pubic ligaments begin to relax under the influence of the hormone relaxin, and the pubic symphyses start to separate. This process can happen up to a week before the onset of parturition, or it may occur as late as only 2 hours before. At the time of the birth this separation should be at least 15 mm, and is often as much as 22 mm.

The delivery of the young takes an average of 30 minutes, with an interval of 3–7 minutes between young. The majority of sows give birth at night.

Complications at parturition

Stillbirths

These account for the majority of losses in guinea pig breeding, and are usually the result of a long and difficult labour and the young are found dead still in their amniotic sacs. There is evidence that feeding sows during gestation on pellets of over 20% protein is one of the factors which causes large fetuses that are stillborn.

Comment. The optimum age for a sow to have her first litter is at 5–6 months, and definitely before she is 10 months old. Between these ages her pelvic bones and muscles stretch easily to allow the passage of young through the birth canal, and this stretching remains permanent for subsequent litters. At 5 months old the pelvis is only partly fused, and fusion occurs over the next 5 months to produce a rigid structure. If the onset of breeding is delayed until the sow is over a year old the pelvic bones are already set and less flexible and dystocia is more common.

Dystocia

This occurs when the young are too large to pass through the pelvic canal or if one of the fetuses is malpresented. Primary uterine inertia appears to be an uncommon cause of dystocia although it may account for some sows close to parturition which are suddenly found dead in the morning despite seeming in good health previously.

Clinical signs. If a sow strains continually for over 20 minutes or fails to produce a young after 2 hours of intermittent straining, dystocia should be considered. If the sow remains in difficulties after this length of time she will rapidly become depressed and she may have a greenish–brown discharge from the vagina.

Careful examination of the cervix is necessary as is an assessment of the degree of separation of the pubic symphyses (which should be 15–20 mm).

Treatment. If there is adequate separation of the symphyses, parturition can be induced by injection of 1–2 iu of oxytocin (Tx 48).

If part of a fetus is presented at the pelvic canal but appears stuck, plenty of lubrication (either Vaseline, liquid paraffin or obstetric lubricant) can be applied and it may then be possible to deliver the fetus using gentle traction. Up to 10 ml of liquid paraffin can be introduced into the uterus via a short catheter or a piece of drip tubing attached to a syringe, this is especially useful if most of the natural lubrication provided by the maternal uterine fluids has been lost and the interior of the uterus has become dry.

Some difficult births, especially those in the breech position can be helped by putting the sow's body under water to assist the contractions.

If parturition does not commence within 15 minutes of an oxytocin injection, or if the fetus is not delivered by other means it will be necessary to proceed with caesarean section.

Comment. One of the major causes of dystocia is a fetal abnormality known as 'bull backed'. This usually arises when mating two roan-coloured cavies together, because of the lethal gene carried by roans. The fetuses are massive and short-backed with the spine curved inwards and the flesh along the back is open. The genetalia are displaced high on the rump, the legs are short and bent and the head is large with the neck in extension. They are always born dead.

Roan × roan matings should be avoided as this lethal gene is also associated with microphthalmia and digestive disorders.

Prevention. Dystocia due to uterine inertia may be associated with a sub-clinical hypocalcaemia and calcium supplementation (Tx 53) once the pubic symphyses begin to separate may prevent this problem.

Premature loss of amniotic fluid

This occurs very occasionally. A sow close to term will suddenly lose her large shape, even to the extent that she looks non-pregnant. This is due to early loss of the amniotic fluid which, if it does not immediately trigger parturition, will lead to fetal death. The sow will subsequently succumb to septicaemia.

Uterine prolapse

This can occur at parturition due to excessive straining, and is therefore often a sequel to dystocia, especially in the young sow. It has also been seen in an aged sow in very poor condition 2 weeks after parturition.

Treatment. This is usually unsuccessful. The uterus can be cleaned and replaced but it often reprolapses as soon as the sow strains to pass faeces. Affected sows are usually in too weak a state to survive surgery and euthanasia should be considered.

Vaginal prolapse

This is not a common condition, but some sows may have a permanent vaginal prolapse. Replacement is unsuccessful, and provided that the prolapse does not compromise the urethral opening it will not cause any problems. It is inadvisable to breed from sows with this condition as problems at parturition are unavoidable.

Post-partum haemorrhage

Some sows may bleed excessively after parturition. In the absence of trauma this has been linked to a vitamin K deficiency as it has been recorded in sows on a diet of dry food and poor hay only. Green foods are the major source of this vitamin and they must be included in the diet. The recommended requirement of vitamin K is 2 mg/kg of feed.

Treatment. Clinical cases are often fatal. Whatever the cause an intramuscular injection of 0.2 ml vitamin K (Konakion) can be tried as this will aid blood clotting.

Mutilation of the young

Guinea pigs never eat their young deliberately. Injuries are only likely to occur during difficult births, especially those in the breech position when the sow may pull at a leg to assist delivery and inadvertantly mutilate the youngster.

Caesarean section

The sooner that dystocia is recognized and caesarean section is carried out the better the chances are of survival of the sow and her litter. However if the sow has already had a long and tiring labour and is depressed and weak her chances of surviving an anaesthetic and surgery are much reduced. In cases where the sow is very weak the operation is best looked upon as a salvage procedure to deliver live young. Baby guinea pigs are born at a very advanced state of development, fully furred and with their eyes open and hand-rearing is often very satisfying. They begin to nibble at solid food as early as their second day and can either be fostered or fed with a dropper (see later).

If, however, the dystocia is recognized early and caesarean section undertaken immediately it can be a successful and satisfying procedure. For details of the anaesthetics and preparation for surgery see Chapter 10.

Surgical procedure. The guinea pig is best placed in dorsal recumbency and the surgery carried out through a midline incision. The uterus should be opened close to its bifurcation and the young and placentas delivered through this incision. This wound should then be closed using an inverting continuous suture of catgut or other absorbable material. Closure of the peritoneum and muscle can be done as one layer, preferably using an interrupted suture pattern. If possible the preferred method of closing the skin is with a sub-cuticular continuous stitch using an absorbable suture (e.g. Vicryl) as the sow will not then have the added stress of returning to the surgery for suture removal, and it also produces a neat wound which does not interfere with the young as they sit under their mother or suckle from her.

Post-operatively the sow should be given an intramuscular injection of 1 unit of oxytocin (Tx 48), 10−15 ml of warmed glucose−saline given subcutaneously (Tx 15), and antibiosis only if the latter is considered necessary. Oral calcium supplementation (Tx 53) for the first 4−5 days after surgery will help prevent the development of post-operative ketosis (see section on pregnancy toxaemia). The sow should be allowed to recover quietly with her young in a warm box and offered glucose water to drink, either from a dish or a dropper. It may be necessary to give the young some supplementary hand-feeding if their mother is weak.

Comment. Sows that have had a caesarean section should not be bred from again as they carry a higher risk of developing complications at subsequent pregnancies.

Complications after parturition

Rejection of the young

Clinical signs. Some mothers, especially after they have experienced a difficult birth, appear terrified of their young and refuse to let them suckle, despite having initially licked them dry.

Treatment. Patient introduction of the young to the sow by gently holding them underneath her and letting her smell them. An intramuscular injection of 1 mg diazepam (Tx 51) will calm the sow and help her adjust to her babies. The sow is best penned in a small box covered with a towel with plenty of nourishing food near the babies whilst she learns to accept them.

Mastitis

Clinical signs. The affected gland may become warm, hard and swollen. In severe cases it may undergo ulceration and necrosis. The sow may become systemically ill.

Treatment. Broad spectrum antibiotics (Tx 1−9) for at least a week usually effect a cure. If ulceration is present the gland must be kept clean and a topical agent such as Dermisol (Tx 25) can be used.

As the causal agents are numerous it may be advisable to run a culture test first so that an appropriate antibiotic can be chosen.

If the affected gland is very hard and painful the application of hot compresses (cotton wool soaked in warm water) will be beneficial. If possible the mammary gland should be stripped frequently and the infected milk expressed. If the sow is fed no greens for a few days this will help decrease her milk production.

Comment. The factors which predispose to the development of this condition are usually environmental, i.e. a poor standard of cleanliness and a build up of faecal contamination in the hutch. It should therefore be possible to prevent its occurrence by improving hygiene and hutch cleanliness. Many bacteria have been isolated from these cases especially *Pseudomonas aeruginosa*, *Pasturella multocida*, *Corynebacterium pyogenes*, *Staphylococcus aureus*, *Streptococcus* spp. and a variety of *Enterobacteriacae*.

Sore nipples

Clinical signs. This may occur if the sow is suckling a large litter. The teats may appear stretched and reddened, but not mastitic. It may also be a problem if the sow's milk supply is sparse as the youngsters suck harder when they try to feed. The sow only has two inguinal mammary glands, and if she is nursing a large litter they are put under a lot of strain.

Treatment. Applying Kamillosan cream (Tx 26, a herbal preparation available from most chemists) several times a day to the affected area will soon relieve the soreness. It is perfectly safe to use this preparation whilst the young are suckling as it causes no harm on ingestion.

If the problem is due to agalactia or poor milk supply the sow can be provided with extra milk by giving her pellets or bran mash which has been soaked in milk or by adding milk to her water bottle.

Comment. Occasionally a sow may possess two or three extra teats. However these teats are generally blind and produce no milk.

Agalactia

Clinical signs. The young have a tucked-up starved appearance. The sow may resent the young suckling from her as her nipples may be sore. This problem is more common if the sow has had a long and difficult labour.

Treatment. Stress must be avoided as this inhibits the flow of milk. The sow and her young should be isolated and kept quiet. The young can be fed a milk preparation by dropper if necessary (see below). The sow can be offered a bran and brown bread mix soaked in milk or alternatively her water bottle can be filled with evaporated milk diluted 1:1 with water. In 2–3 days her young will also be drinking from this bottle and the frequency of hand-supplementation can be reduced.

Injections of oxytocin soon after birth to improve milk let-down are not recommended as the stress they produce outweighs their beneficial effect.

Comment. Immediately after parturition milk let-down is under the control of oxytocin which is released from the posterior pituitary following stimulation of the nipple during suckling and also from stimulus to the cervix as a fetus passes through the birth canal. The practice of eating the placentas is also a stimulus for milk production. For the remainder of lactation, milk secretion is under the control of prolactin, a hormone whose release is triggered by stimulation of the nipple during suckling. Therefore if the young are totally hand-reared it is unlikely that the sow will produce much milk as the stimulus for milk secretion is lost. However, if a sow is unstressed and well fed, her milk flow should return and it may only be necessary to supplement the young for the first 24 hours.

It is not necessary to hand-feed the young soon after birth as they may not become hungry for the first 12 hours, during which time the sow may have settled down and begun producing milk.

Eclampsia

Clinical signs. This is a rare condition but has been seen in older sows up to 7 days after parturition especially if suckling a large litter. The sow becomes suddenly depressed and twitches. In later stages she goes into fits. Ketosis will also produce similar symptoms.

Treatment. An intraperitoneal injection of 5 ml of 10% calcium solution can be attempted, but it is unlikely to be successful in later stages of this condition.

Comment. During lactation it is advisable to feed a variety of calcium-rich food. Carrots, beetroot and watercress are all good sources of calcium, although the latter must be fed sparingly. Milk thistle (sow thistle) is also a useful supplement during lactation. Calcium supplementation (Tx 53) can be given to the sow during the last week of gestation and first week of lactation.

Skin complaints

Sows quite commonly develop raw patches on their rumps and ventral abdomens after birth. They may also develop a bare patch in the centre of their backs after parturition, known as a 'post-natal sore' (see Chapter 1). Hair loss is also common in the last trimester of pregnancy when the metabolic demands on the sow are high.

Orphans

As they are born at such an advanced stage of development orphans have a good chance of survival. The young start picking at solid food and hay as early as the second day and babies orphaned at 3 days old have been known to survive given no supplementation.

It is possible to use a foster mother if one is available, indeed if two or more nursing females are penned together their young may steal feeds from the other mothers.

If no foster mother is available the orphans can be reared on a suitable milk replacer fed through a dropper (e.g. Welpi or Sherley's Lactol). The powder should be mixed with water to a consistency that can run through a dropper, and initially they should be fed every 2 hours. They will probably take 1−2 ml of milk per feed during the first few days, and once they are 5 days old, and beginning to nibble at solid food, they need only be fed 4-hourly and at this stage they may take as much as 3 ml at one feed. However hand-feeding need not be started until the young are 12 hours old as they will not become hungry until then.

The milky mixture can also be mixed with brown bread in a dish so that they can learn to feed themselves. Minced carrot, beetroot and soaked pellets can also be offered in the early days, but they will soon nibble at adult food. If no foster mother with milk is available it is a good idea to keep them with an adult guinea pig who can provide them with warmth and companionship. The baby guinea pigs will also copy the adult and soon start nibbling at solids. Once the young are drinking from the water bottle attached to the cage door this can be filled with evaporated milk diluted 1 : 1 with water.

As with the hand-rearing of any animal, care must be taken not to force the milk into the mouth in order to avoid causing inhalation pneumonia.

After each feed, it is important to clean their faces and to stimulate them to pass urine and faeces by stroking their lower abdomens with a piece of damp cotton wool.

An alternative recipe for a milk replacer that the author uses is evaporated milk diluted 1 : 2 with cooled boiled water and thickened with Farex to a consistency that will run through a dropper. A drop of Abidec (Tx 52, vitamin drops available from the chemist, containing vitamins A, B, C and D) is added to one feed of the day.

Comment. The composition of guinea pig milk is:
- 3.9% fat.
- 8.1% protein.
- 3% lactose.

The composition of cows milk is:
- 3.8% fat.

- 3.3% protein.
- 4.7% lactose.

Thus evaporated milk is a close approximation, and as the young are soon nibbling at concentrates they can easily make up the protein deficit.

It is important to encourage the orphans to eat solid foods as early as possible as a high percentage of orphans which receive too much milk replacer develop cataracts and become blind. The development of cataracts is thought to be associated with the intake of too many complex sugars which are dissimilar to those found in natural guinea pig milk.

Fostering

A suitable foster mother is one with a small litter of 2−3 days old. She should be put in a small box and her babies removed. The orphans should then be rubbed with the other young so that they all smell alike. Alternatively a metholated vapour rub (e.g. Vick) can be dabbed under the mothers chin and on all the babies so that all different smells are eradicated. The orphans can then be introduced to the foster mother and provided they are accepted the rest of the litter can be returned an hour later.

Nursing guinea pigs also make ideal foster parents for orphan chinchillas. The author has also successfully hand-reared a chinchilla with the help of a sow which had never had a litter, yet she instinctively took over every other aspect of caring for the orphan apart from the feeding.

2.4   Infertility

The boar

Often it is the very large boars that are sterile. To check the boar, it is necessary to extrude his penis by pushing in on his abdomen just cranial to his genitalia. At the end of a normal penis there are two horns or prongs. These should be of equal length, but if one is missing or they are of differing lengths the boar will be sterile. Unfortunately some boars with normal looking genitalia can also be sterile.

If the boar is not given his first opportunity to mate before he is a year old, his sex drive will diminish rapidly. For this reason it is advisable to put a boar with his first sow when he is 4–5 months old. Overshowing will also lead to decreased sex drive.

Preputial prolapse

In adult boars the prepuce may stretch and this leads to the penis not being fully encased within the body, but up to 0.4 cm may be left outside and the prepuce falls into folds around it. Particles of food, hay and straw collect in the folds and cause irritation and infection. Such boars often become sterile.

Treatment. The penis and prepuce must be examined carefully, and if necessary cleaned with a weak saline solution (Tx 59) and topical anti-bacterial cream applied (e.g. Tx 25, Dermisol). This must be applied sparingly as the boar is likely inadvertantly to ingest some when he collects his caecal faeces to redigest.

Preputial infections

These usually occur secondarily to foreign bodies such as grass seeds or sawdust becoming lodged in the prepuce. These may also lead to an inability to copulate. Preputial dermatitis may lead to a swelling of the prepuce and perineum.

Treatment. Removal of any foreign bodies and treatment of the infection. A topical preparation may be sufficient for this purpose (Tx 25–28).

Comment. Sawdust may also block the vagina of the female and lead to an inability of the male to achieve copulation. For this reason using sawdust as a bedding material should be discouraged, and the use of woodshavings recommended instead.

The sow

A sow may be naturally barren or she may become temporarily unable to conceive if she is in poor condition and underweight. A sow may become barren after a history of miscarriages or abortions. If she has recovered from an attack of cystitis she may also become infertile.

Many sows will just stop breeding once they reach 3−5 years of age.

Treatment of both sexes

It is impossible to cure those that are naturally sterile and these should be removed from the breeding programme.

1   By improving the condition of the breeding sows their ability to conceive should return. It is important that litters are planned to coincide with maximum availability of greenstuff, i.e. March− September. It is therefore best to begin pairing the sows and boars in January.

2   Each sow should be allowed adequate time to rest and regain her strength between litters (at least a month). No sow should have more than two or three litters a year.

3   Addition of a little wheatgerm oil to the food daily may improve fertility. Wheatgerm consists almost entirely of vitamin E. A lack of adequate vitamin E leads to degeneration of the seminiferous tubules in the male.

4   There should be adequate provision of good hay, as although the cavy does not build a nest it does like to burrow. Reproductive performance has been shown to decrease in the absence of hay.

5   If the environmental temperature is too high this may lead to infertility. This phenomenon is seen during very hot summers. The recommendations for optimum temperature and humidity are:
- Room temperature: 20−22°C (68−72°F).
- Humidity: 45−65%.

6   It is important that the breeding hutches receive plenty of light. Both inadequate lighting and shortened daylight hours lead to infertility.

Comment. Guinea pigs are polyoestrus and come into season all the year round. At the time of ovulation the level of oestrogen in their serum rises to a maximum. Ovulation occurs when this coincides with a surge of a second hormone, luteinizing hormone (LH). The latter is released from the anterior pituitary under the control of GnRH (gonadotrophin-releasing factor) from the hypothalamus.

The LH surge is subject to control by a daily rhythm. The GnRH, neurones are influenced by a neural signal carrying information about light/dark cycles from the retina. Thus, if the breeding stock are kept in poor light there will be insufficient stimulus for this sequence of hormone release and therefore no trigger for ovulation.

Therefore, by improving the lighting to the breeding quarters and, if necessary, using artificial lighting to create the required 10–12 hours of light per day it should be possible to provide the correct environmental stimuli necessary for this sequence of hormonal events leading to ovulation.

The hormonal control of gonadal activity in the male is constant, and not cyclical as in the female. However, environmental factors play just as important a role in governing the reproductive activity of the male and thus the above comments about infertility apply equally to both sexes.

It is best not to breed from sows or boars which take a long time to mate successfully as their offspring are likely to inherit the same problems.

Cystic ovaries

The incidence of this condition in guinea pigs is unknown but it may be an important contributing factor to sow infertility or her inability to carry a litter to term.

The ovary can contain multiple fluid-filled cysts up to 1 cm in diameter, and the condition is usually bilateral.

Treatment. None as the condition is usually only discovered post-mortem.

Metritis

Mild cases may only result in a failure to become pregnant. More severe cases may occur after abortion or difficult births and are usually fatal. Some cases have been associated with *Bordetella* infection.

Vaginal discharge

This must not be confused with the normal opaque creamy coloured urine which may be seen by the genitalia. A vaginal discharge accompanied by infertility is suggestive of metritis.

Treatment. A vaginal swab should be taken for culture and sensitivity tests. A suitable broad-spectrum antibiotic can then be used to treat the infection (Tx 1–9).

Comment. Haemolytic streptococci are commonly implicated as a cause of this condition.

Castration

The inguinal canal of the male guinea pig remains open throughout life, and there is therefore an increased risk of a prolapse of abdominal contents after castration. In times of stress (e.g. anaesthesia) the male guinea pig is able to withdraw his testes completely into the abdomen.

Surgical procedure. A skin incision should be made in the scrotum at either side of the penis. The tunic should then be incised and the testicle can be grasped. Gentle traction will reveal the spermatic cord and a mass of fat. A ligature should be placed around the cord below the mass of fat and to include the tunic. The spermatic cord can then be cut and the skin closed. The preferred method of skin closure is to use a sub-cuticular stitch with an absorbable suture material as this avoids the stress of suture removal.

3/ The Urinary System

3.1 Anatomy

The guinea pig has two kidneys, the right kidney being placed further forward in the body than the left. A ureter runs from each renal pelvis to enter the bladder (see Fig. 3.1). A single urethra runs from the bladder to the urethral opening.

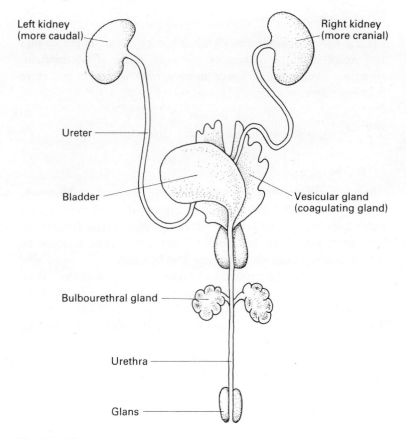

Fig. 3.1 The urinary tract.

The male urethra is longer and less distendable than that of the female and as it passes from the bladder to the urethral opening it is closely associated with the vesicular (coagulating) gland, the prostate and the bulbourethral gland.

3.2 Physiology

Normal guinea pig urine is opaque and creamy yellow in colour. It is alkaline and has a normal pH of 9. The urine occasionally contains crystals of ammonium phosphate and calcium carbonate. This crystaluria accounts for a build up of scale in the hutches which can easily be removed by cleaning with a weak acid solution.

Urinary tract disorders

Little is known about the incidence of kidney disease in guinea pigs and many definitive diagnoses are only made at postmortem. However, symptoms of lower urinary tract disorders are more frequently seen in general practice.

3.3 Symptoms of urinary tract disorders

Polydipsia

The average water intake of a guinea pig is 10 ml/100 g. However, this is very variable and if the diet consists of foods with a high water content, e.g. lettuce and other succulent green foods, very little extra water will be drunk. Water intake does increase by varying amounts during pregnancy and lactation.

Polydipsia can be expected to occur in cases of chronic renal failure and diabetes. Polydipsia accompanied by a large abdominal swelling has been seen in a case of hydronephrosis of both kidneys. The affected individual was not ill but was euthanased when the swelling became severe.

A diet consisting of a large amount of dandelions, which induce diuresis, will lead to a resultant transient polydipsia.

Polyuria

The average urinary output of an adult is 20−25 ml per day.

Polyuria is only seen as a consequence of polydipsia, or when eating large quantities of foods with diuretic properties (e.g. dandelions). Excess urine output may lead to urine scalding which can present a problem in both sexes, and this is seen clinically as a moist dermatitis around the genitals ventrally in the sow, and around the rump in the male.

This consequent urine scalding can be treated with topical applications of Dermisol or Vetsovate twice daily (Tx 25 or 28). The affected area can be protected with Vaseline or a resistant barrier cream such as zinc and castor oil cream.

Guinea pigs which are prone to the development of this condition should be kept on an absorbent bedding such as newspaper and woodshavings to minimize the problem of urine soaking their coats.

Haematuria ('bloody urine')

Passing blood in the urine is a fairly common complaint, and is seen equally frequently in boars and sows.

Clinical signs. The affected animal is often still in good health, or may exhibit pain during urination, by arching its back and crying.

Causes of haematuria. These include:
1 Cystitis. If cystitis is suspected a course of broad-spectrum antibiotics can be given for 7 days; ones that are commonly used are sulphamezathine or Tribrissen (Tx 7 and 9). A human preparation of nitrofurantoin (Tx 6) has also been successful at a dose of 50 mg a day for 3 days.

Once a sow has had an attack of cystitis she may become infertile.
2 Neoplasia. Unfortunately the passing of bloody urine is frequently associated with tumours of the bladder or uterus. If the cavy is still bright, eating and not in severe discomfort, supportive measures can be instituted (B vitamins and iron-rich foods such as spinach, grass and dandelions). If there is severe discomfort euthanasia is the kindest option.
3 Urolithiasis. See below.

True haematuria must be differentiated from the red-coloured urine produced by guinea pigs on a diet consisting of large quantities of beetroot.

Crystaluria

The urine is naturally alkaline and may contain phosphate and carbonate crystals. These generally cause no problems but may form as a scale around the cage. However, together with other predisposing factors such as low water intake these crystals may form larger calculi.

Occlusion of the penile urethra

Coagulum from the vesicular glands may block the terminal portion of the urethra and lead to a secondary cystitis.

Clinical signs. Pain on urination is a common feature. Haematuria associated with the secondary cystitis may also be evident.

Treatment. Cleansing of the affected area, and broad-spectrum antibiotics if there is a concurrent cystitis (Tx 1−9).

Urolithiasis

The formation of stones is more common in the boar as his urethra is longer and less distendable than that of the sow. Normal urine may contain small calculi and under certain circumstances these may form larger stones. In older males, concretions are found in the urethra and in the prepuce and these in part are the result of congealed ejaculum and crystals which readily becomes infected with *Pseudomonas aeruginosa*, *Proteus* and *Escherichia coli*.

If just a few stones are present in the urinary tract they may only partially obstruct the urinary flow, and over a period of time the resultant back pressure on the kidneys may cause a progressive hydronephrosis.

Clinical signs. These are variable. In mild cases they may be absent whilst more severely affected individuals may exhibit dysuria or anuria (seen as a hunched posture and crying when attempting to urinate), haematuria, anorexia and listlessness.

The stones may be palpable and occasionally they can be felt as a hard lump inside the prepuce. They will also be evident on radiographs.

Treatment. (1) Surgical removal from the bladder and subsequent antibiotic treatment has been reported to be successful. (2) Stones present inside the sheath can be removed manually by extruding the penis. (3) Small calculi may be dissolved if the urine is acidified, however, guinea pigs do have difficulty in removing an acid load. Some acidification of the urine can be achieved by feeding more of foods with a high acid content, e.g. apple and beetroot.

Comment. The aetiology of stone formation is unclear. However, predisposing factors include a low water intake, nutritional imbalances and bacterial infections. There also seems to be an inherited disposition to their development.

Hydronephrosis

One or both kidneys may become cystic and fluid-filled.

Clinical signs. Polydipsia and palpable abdominal swellings. In the early stages, the guinea pig remains well but as the condition progresses other signs associated with chronic renal failure become apparent. This condition is usually seen in guinea pigs over the age of 4 years.

Pathology. The affected kidney has most of its normal structure replaced and becomes a fluid-filled sac with a rim of atrophied parenchyma. When a single kidney becomes hydronephrotic the other kidney can function alone. However, chronic renal failure will occur if the other kidney also becomes affected. Thus in postmortem examinations the condition is often found to be bilateral.

Acute renal failure

This is an infrequent but fatal condition in guinea pigs. However, it may occur due to oxalic acid poisoning which may result from the ingestion of large amounts of beetroot, spinach or dock leaves once the stems have turned woody as all of these contain oxalic acid.

Clinical signs before death include depression, salivation and muscle tremors. Numerous crystals of calcium oxalate precipitate out in the kidney and urinary tract.

Chronic renal failure

Clinical signs. Chronic renal disease is insidious in onset and initially the only sign may be polydipsia. As the disease progresses there may be a period of anorexia and depression, diarrhoea, then collapse and death.

Pathology. The affected kidneys are smaller in size and much of their parenchyma is replaced with fibrous tissue ('end-stage' kidneys). If the renal failure is as a result of progressive hydronephrosis, the normal parenchyma will be replaced by a thin-walled sac which will be full of fluid.

Diabetes

Clinical signs. Polydipsia and weight loss despite maintaining a good appetite. Some individuals may also develop cataracts.

Diagnosis. Blood glucose can be determined from a drop of blood obtained by overclipping a toenail. Normal values lie between 60 and 125 mg/100 ml (3−7 mmol/litre).

4/ The Respiratory System

4.1 Anatomy and physiology

Guinea pigs possess a normal mammalian respiratory system with no specific peculiarities. The healthy guinea pig will only breath through its nose and therefore mouth breathing is a sign of respiratory distress.

They are particularly susceptible to bronchospasm if ether is used as an anaesthetic agent and for this reason it is not recommended.

4.2 Symptoms of respiratory disorders

Sneezing

All guinea pigs sneeze occasionally, especially if they are exposed to dusty food or hay. Guinea pigs bedded on fine sawdust are also inclined to sneeze frequently. Sneezing is their body's natural defence mechanism for keeping their nasal passages clear. However, if the sneezing becomes more frequent or it is accompanied by a mucopurulent or haemopurulent discharge it may be a symptom of a more serious disease condition.

Epistaxis

Bleeding from the nose may be a symptom of vitamin K deficiency. This can arise if the diet consists of dry food and poor hay only as the major source of this vitamin is from greenstuffs.

Epistaxis may also be present after trauma, especially if the guinea pig has fallen on its head.

Nasal discharge

A mucopurulent discharge is usually a symptom of upper or lower respiratory tract infection. However, this must not be confused with a normal milky fluid which is occasionally exuded from the nose and eyes as part of the natural grooming process.

Coughing

As with sneezing, all guinea pigs will cough occasionally and this need not be related to a pathological condition but is assumed to be a part of the body's natural defence mechanism.

Snuffles

Certain types of guinea pig, especially those with short noses, may snuffle as they breathe. This problem may be present from birth and these youngsters are more prone to developing respiratory disease later. These guinea pigs encounter similar problems to those of the brachycephalic breeds of dog.

Ruttling

This term describes a rough sounding wheezy type of breathing made by guinea pigs (râles). It is often a symptom of an infectious disease condition, however, it may present unassociated with a disease process. The origin of this sound is unclear.

4.3 Respiratory infections

Predisposing factors. A change in environmental temperature, humidity or ventilation. Ammonia produced as a consequence of a build up of dirty litter will also weaken the resistance of the respiratory tract to infection. Other factors include a sudden diet change, diets low in vitamin C and overcrowded housing. The young, old and pregnant are the most susceptible groups for developing respiratory disease.

Pneumonia

Clinical signs. The symptoms of pneumonia are similar regardless of the causative agent and include dyspnoea, ruttling, sneezing accompanied by a nasal discharge and coughing. The affected guinea pig adopts a tucked-up appearance, becomes depressed and anorexic and, if left untreated, will die. In some cases the infection progresses to the middle and inner ear causing torticollis. Even with treatment the outcome can be fatal.

This condition can be caused by numerous bacterial and viral agents. The most common of these is *Bordetella bronchiseptica*, but others include *Streptococcus zooepidemicus* (see Chapter 7), *Streptococcus pneumoniae*, *Klebsiella pneumoniae*, *Pseudomonas aeruginosa* and *Pasturella* spp.

Bordetella and *Streptococcus pneumoniae* may also cause uterine infections and abortion, either as a separate entity or as part of a more generalized infection.

Diagnosis. Isolation of the causal agent from a culture of tracheal exudate.

Pathology. At post-mortem *Bordetella* infections reveal consolidation of a lobe of lung, accompanied by signs of a prurulent bronchitis, suppuration, exudation and haemorrhage. *Streptococcus* infections produce seroprurulent and fibrinoprurulent lesions of the pleural cavity, lungs, pericardium and occasionally the peritoneum. In cases of sudden death in pregnant sows abscesses may be present in the uterine wall.

Treatment. Broad-spectrum antibiotics, e.g. a trimethoprim−sulphonamide combination (Tx 9) or sulphamezathine (Tx 7). However, antibiotics may not eliminate the carrier state. In the case of *Streptococcus zooepidemicus* the use of a cephalosporin (Tx 2) is recommended. If the lungs are very congested concurrent treatment with a diuretic (e.g. frusemide − Lasix 5% solution − at a dose rate of 0.1 ml given by intramuscular injection) is recommended.

The affected guinea pig must be isolated in a warm, clean and well-ventilated environment. A little mentholated vapour rub (e.g. Vick) can be applied around the hutch and this will help clear the nasal passages. Alternatively Eucalyptus oil can be used for the same purpose. Some Vick can also be dabbed on the chest or on the inside of the forelegs where the skin is bare. If the guinea pig is anorexic, an appetite stimulant such as Vetrumex can be given mixed with some water and 2−3 drops of Abidec vitamins. An old remedy for colds and asthma was to feed coltsfoot, and if this is available it can be included in the guinea pig's diet.

Increasing the water vapour content of the environment by using the steam from a boiling kettle, or by placing the individual in the bathroom will help soothe the nasal passages and loosen the mucus in the bronchi.

Epidemiology. This may include the following conditions.

1 *Bordetella bronchiseptica* may be introduced via symptomless carriers of other species, e.g. dogs, cats and rabbits, and care must be taken if these species are brought into close contact with guinea pigs. Outbreaks of *Bordetella* are precipitated by stress. The incubation period is 3−7 days.

2 *Streptococcus pneumoniae* is spread by direct or indirect (aerosol) routes. Some individuals may exist as symptomless carriers and carry the organism in their upper respiratory tract.

Prevention. The environmental factors should be kept constant. Where possible the room temperature should be 20−22°C, and the relative humidity 45−65%. The hutches should be cleaned regularly to prevent the accumulation of ammonia. The ventilation should be good, but the caviary must be free from draughts.

Vaccination using an autogenous formalin killed bacterin given intramuscularly has been described. This gives adequate protection for 4−6 months, and its use was successful in eliminating the carrier state from an affected colony. Porcine *Bordetella* bacterins will also protect cavies against fatal pneumonias.

Non-infectious ruttling

The aetiology of this is unclear. Guinea pigs of the short-nosed type seem more prone to developing abnormal respiratory sounds. It is more common in winter when the hay and dry food are more dusty. Other causes that have been suggested are sawdust, high pollen counts, and stress in highly strung individuals. In the cases associated with hay and pollen the likely mechanism is the development of an allergic type bronchitis, which may clear once the allergen has been eliminated.

This condition has also been referred to as 'beetroot ruttle' in the past but no link between the two has been made.

Clinical signs. The respiratory sounds become wheezy and rough sounding. In comparison with infectious conditions the guinea pig remains otherwise healthy and eats well.

Treatment. A 5-day course of sulphamezathine (Tx 7) can be given but some cases may never be completely cured.

5/ The Digestive System

5.1 Anatomy

The anatomy of the digestive tract is displayed in Fig. 5.1. In contrast to other rodents the guinea pig has a very long colon, which accounts for 60% of the length of its intestines. It also has a

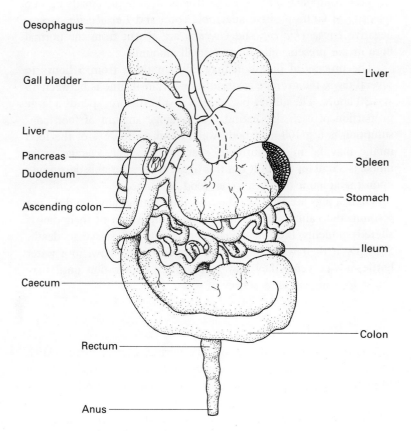

Oesophagus

Gall bladder

Liver

Pancreas

Duodenum

Ascending colon

Caecum

Rectum

Anus

Liver

Spleen

Stomach

Ileum

Colon

Fig. 5.1 The digestive tract.

large caecum for digestion of cellulose, a feature which is typical of a herbivore. The wall of this organ is thin and it contains numerous lateral pouches which further increase its capacity with the result that the caecum is able to contain up to 65% of the gastrointestinal contents at any one time.

The stomach is non-glandular and the spleen is closely associated to it and is relatively broad. The female's spleen is significantly larger and heavier than that of the male.

5.2 Physiology

The intestinal tract contains large numbers of non-pathogenic protozoa and *Candida albicans* is also present in normal gut flora. The bacterial component of normal gastrointestinal flora is made up of a majority of Gram-positive anaerobic cocci and *Lactobacilli*. Gram-negative *Escherichia coli* and *Coccidia* are absent from the normal flora or are present only in very small amounts.

The process of digestion may take anything from 5 hours to several days; the average gastrointestinal transit time is between 13 and 30 hours. The guinea pig, typical of a herbivore, spends a large proportion of each day eating. The average amount of food consumption is 6 g/100 g of body weight and up to 75% of the food intake may be in the form of concentrates. The average water intake is 85 ml for an adult but this figure is very variable depending upon the amount of moist green food consumed.

Guinea pigs are very fastidious in their eating habits and do not accommodate alterations easily. If the composition of their diet is altered suddenly they may just stop eating and starve to death. Similarly if their water supply is changed from a bowl to a water bottle or vice versa they may suffer water deprivation until they adjust to using the new source of water.

Coprophagia

The eating of its own droppings is a normal part of the digestive process. The guinea pig selectively eats the smaller moist droppings taking them directly from the anus. These lighter and softer faeces are caecal faeces and contain the important B-complex vitamins which are formed by bacterial flora in the caecum. By redigesting these faeces the cavy satisfies its need for B vitamins. Young guinea pigs will also be seen eating their mother's droppings. In this way the young guinea pigs populate their guts with a balanced bacterial flora before weaning.

Impaction of the rectum

Clinical signs. This is seen as a hard swelling inside the anus of older boars. The muscles of the anus become stretched and the inside of the rectum becomes impacted with the softer and moister caecal faeces. The boar may start to lose condition if he is unable to remove and redigest these caecal faeces. He is often still able to pass the harder droppings past the impaction.

Treatment. Petroleum jelly (Vaseline) or olive oil can be smeared inside the anus and the mass of faeces can be squeezed out manually. Once this condition develops in a boar he will need to be cleared out on a weekly basis. If the boar is not redigesting any caecal faeces he may also require supplementation with a vitamin B complex.

Diarrhoea (scours)

The guinea pig is unable to vomit so anything that it ingests has to pass through the digestive tract. The majority of diarrhoea cases result from sudden dietary changes or from the ingestion of poor quality foodstuffs. However if it is seen as an enzootic problem infectious causes must be considered. It is also seen as a symptom in more generalized disease conditions such as chronic kidney or liver failure.

Infectious causes of diarrhoea

Salmonella

The causal agents are usually *Salmonella typhimurium* or *Salmonella enteriditis*. The disease generally enters the caviary via carrier mice and rats which may contaminate the food and hay.

Clinical signs. Acute enteritis which may be haemorrhagic; also sudden deaths (septicaemia), abortions, and in chronic cases weight loss and poor condition. The disease will spread rapidly through the caviary.

Pathology. At post-mortem there is splenic enlargement and focal necrosis of this organ and the liver which may also be enlarged. There will also be hyperaemia of the intestines accompanied by mesenteric lymph node enlargement. In per-acute cases splenic enlargement may be the only feature and there are no lesions in carrier animals.

Diagnosis. Isolation of *Salmonella* spp. in faecal samples.

Treatment. Affected animals should be destroyed and preferably disposed of by burning as *Salmonella* is zoonotic. Healthy guinea pigs should be removed from the affected premises and housed separately elsewhere. All premises and feeding and drinking utensils should be thoroughly disinfected, and any bedding and hay should be burnt.

Chloramphenicol (Tx 3) at a dose of $20-55$ mg/kg orally three times a day or 6.5 mg/kg injected intramuscularly twice daily will effect some cures but its use is very likely to produce resistant strains and perpetuate the carrier state which is an undesirable consequence.

Comment. Chronic cases and those which recover are likely to become carriers of *Salmonella* and they should also be destroyed to prevent further outbreaks of this disease.

Considering the public health risk of this disease it is recommended to depopulate the caviary completely rather than risk perpetuating the disease in its carrier state.

Yersinia (pseudotuberculosis)

Clinical signs. Both acute and chronic forms of this disease are recognized. The acute form causes septicaemia and death within 48 hours. The more chronic form causes a longer period of diarrhoea and weight loss, and occasionally dyspnoea and coughing, often culminating in death after $3-4$ weeks. During this period, any young of the affected guinea pig may become congenitally or neonatally affected. In an emaciated guinea pig the enlarged mesenteric lymph nodes can often be palpated through the abdomen.

In some cases the infection may be contained in the cervical lymph nodes, and this must be differentiated from abscesses and cervical lymphadenitis (see Chapters 1 and 7). In such cases the condition is not usually fatal.

Diagnosis. Culture of *Yersinia pseudotuberculosis* from blood or lymph nodes.

Pathology. Nodular, caseous lesions in the mesenteric lymph nodes, and focal necrosis of the liver and spleen. There may also be lesions in the lungs and pleura.

Treatment. Like *Salmonella* this condition is zoonotic. Affected individuals must be destroyed; all premises and utensils well disinfected.

Comment. The disease is transmitted to guinea pigs via wild birds and rodents which contaminate their green foods. Any green foods should be washed before being fed to guinea pigs. Once it is endemic in a breeding population more chronic forms are seen, and in some cases the infection is passed vertically in the milk.

Clostridia

Clostridia spp. are normally present in small numbers in the large intestine. In certain circumstances (e.g. during antibiotic administration) they are able to proliferate and cause a fatal enterotoxaemia.

Clinical signs. An acute onset of profuse diarrhoea, either green—brown or watery, accompanied by other signs of depression, bloat, abdominal pain and a fetid odour.

Diagnosis. At post-mortem there are signs of a haemorrhagic enteritis, and the gut lumen contains green—brown mucoid material.

Clostridial species can be cultured from the lumen of affected portions of intestine.

Treatment. None available — the condition is fatal.

Enteropathies of unknown origin

A per-acute necrosis of the mucosa of the caecum and large intestine leading to sudden death has been reported.

Escherichia coli is not a normal inhabitant of the gastrointestinal tract and if it is isolated in a case of enteritis it is usually of significance.

Parasitic causes of diarrhoea

Parasitic enteritis is rarely a problem in guinea pigs.

Nematodes

The only nematode which affects guinea pigs is *Paraspidodera uncinata* and infection is generally associated with guinea pigs housed in outdoor runs. Heavy infestations may cause enteritis. *Paraspidodera* usually resides in the caecum and the adult is 11−28 mm long.

Treatment. Thiabendazole at a rate of 100 mg/kg given orally or piperazine (Tx 40) at a dilution of 3 mg/ml in the drinking water.

Protozoa

A large number of protozoa can be carried but these are not usually pathogenic with the exception of *Coccidia* (see below). Of the non-pathogenic species *Trichomonas* and *Entamoeba* spp. are the most frequently isolated.

Complications due to these organisms are generally associated with poor husbandry or severe debilitation from other causes. Sporadic deaths preceded by a short period (3−8 hours) of diarrhoea have been seen in association with a large burden of *Trichomonas* spp. in guinea pigs housed on deep straw litter.

Treatment. Metronidazole (Tx 39, Flagyl) at a dose of 20 mg/kg diluted in the drinking water for 10 days.

Cestoda

Infection due to *Cestoda* is also very infrequent but the guinea pig may act as an alternative host to *Cestoda* which normally use other rodents as their hosts, such as *Hymenolepis* spp., *Taenia crassicollis* and *Echinococcus granulosus*.

Heavy doses of these tapeworms may cause enteritis, intestinal obstruction or retarded growth.

Treatment. Praziquantal (Tx 41, Droncit Bayer) at a dose of 5−10 mg/kg orally or 5 mg/kg by subcutaneous injection.

Cryptosporidium

This has been implicated as a cause of diarrhoea, weight loss and death in young animals but is unlikely to be a problem unless the guinea pig is immunocompromised.

Coccidiosis

Eimeria caviae is the coccidial species recognized in guinea pigs, and infection is usually contracted by the ingestion of contaminated food. It is, however, a very infrequent problem in the domestic guinea pig.

Guinea pigs may become infected with other *Coccidia* spp. if they are in contact with rabbits.

Clinical signs. The droppings are slimy in appearance and contain blood. Affected individuals look generally unthrifty and youngsters fail to gain weight.

Diagnosis. Oocytes are present in the faeces and they may be seen on microscopic examination of the supernatant layer of faecal matter after flotation or on examination of a wet mount prepared directly from the intestinal contents.

Pathology. At post-mortem petichial haemorrhages and greyish-white nodules are present in the wall of the colon.

Treatment. Sulphamezathine (Tx 42) is given to affected guinea pigs for 5 days. Cleanliness is essential and if possible the guinea pigs should be housed on wire flooring to prevent the incidence of reinfection. Oocysts which are present in the hutch can be destroyed by cleaning with a 1% ammonia solution.

Comment. The presence of oocysts of *Eimeria caviae* does not necessarily mean that it is the primary pathogen in a case of diarrhoea.

Ascaridae

Ascaridae are not a natural parasite of guinea pigs but they may occur if the cavy is grazing on grass which has been contaminated with dog or cat faeces.

Clinical signs. Weight loss and unthriftiness, diarrhoea and occasionally signs of intestinal obstruction.

Treatment. Oral administration of fenbendazole at a dose rate of 100 mg/kg as a single dose.

Non-infectious causes of diarrhoea

Dietary

This is a relatively common cause of diarrhoea which affects individuals in the caviary rather than causing a disease of zootic proportions.

Sudden change of diet. This often occurs in spring when there is a sudden increase in the availability of greenstuffs and the temptation is to overfeed rather than to reintroduce green foods slowly and carefully.

Grass clippings. These are one of the major offenders for causing scours as they rapidly overheat. They should only be fed immediately after they have been cut and any that are uneaten after a few hours should be removed.

Plants with a laxative action. If large quantities of these green foods are fed together this will result in diarrhoea. Such plants include groundsel and dandelions. They should be fed in balance with plants with an astringent action such as shepherd's purse, bramble leaves, and young dock leaves.

Mouldy or frosted food. Care must be taken when collecting wild greens from the hedgerows, especially in late summer, to ensure that there is no white mould on the underside of the leaves as this will cause a mucoid enteritis.

Roots must be completely thawed before they are fed if they have been picked when the ground is frozen, and greens covered in frost should not be fed.

Similarly food which has been taken from the refrigerator should not be fed immediately, but allowed to warm a little first. Fresh food remaining in the hutch at night should be removed during the cold weather as it is likely to freeze overnight.

The feeding of frosted food will damage the lining of the stomach wall causing ulceration and subsequent diarrhoea.

Mouldy hay may contain fungal species, notably *Absidia ramosa* and *A. corymbifera*. These may cause a transient localized reaction in the mesenteric lymph nodes and often a profuse diarrhoea. The fungi may also colonize other organs such as the kidneys and spleen with fatal consequences.

Cereals, particularly maize, may become contaminated with fungal spores of *Aspergillus flavus*, and ingestion of these will cause a fatal aphlatoxicosis.

Clinical signs. Although the droppings are loose the guinea pig is still bright in the early stages, and usually continues to eat normally. If the condition is allowed to progress unattended the guinea pig may become dull, depressed and anorexic.

Treatment. All green food must be removed from the diet and the guinea pig fed solely on good hay and dry food. Astringents such as bramble leaves (with the thorns removed) and shepherd's purse can be fed. Arrowroot, either as crumbled biscuits or in its dry form mixed with water is another useful astringent.

Some breeders recommend feeding a bran mash soaked in water to which a little vitamin C has been added instead of the dry food. If the guinea pig's normal diet includes a molasses-enriched dry mix this should certainly be replaced with bran as the molasses will perpetuate the diarrhoea. Plenty of water should be given and in some instances giving diluted liquid Lectade will be beneficial.

If the affected animal is severely dehydrated the subcutaneous administration of warmed glucose−saline (Tx 15) or electrolyte solution (Hartmann's) may be beneficial.

Other preparations which can be used are an infant diarrhoea preparation KLN (Tx 22, available from chemists) or an antibiotic and kaolin preparation (Tx 24, Neosulphentrin suspension, Willows Francis). 3–4 drops of KLN can be given via a dropper or on a teaspoon three times a day.

Sulphamezathine 33% (Tx 7) diluted 1:1 with water to 16.5% strength can be given at a dose of 3 ml three times a day for a maximum of 5 days.

If the guinea pig has become anorexic a useful appetite stimulant is Vetrumex (Tx 13), a preparation which is formulated for cattle to replace their gut's natural bacterial flora. 0.25–0.5 of a teaspoonful can be mixed with a little water and rosehip syrup (source of vitamin C) and this dose can be given daily.

An alternative method of repopulating the affected guinea pig's gut with natural bacterial flora is to feed it fresh droppings from a healthy guinea pig.

Once a guinea pig has recovered a normal diet can be reintroduced very slowly over the following 3–4 weeks, but it may take several more weeks for the guinea pig to regain its former condition.

Antibiotic-induced diarrhoea

The administration of certain antibiotics alters the gut flora in such a way that it allows the intestines to become colonized with *Clostridium* spp. This bacterial proliferation takes place mainly in the caecum. These bacteria produce enterotoxins and cause a fatal enteritis and diarrhoea. The most toxic drugs appear to be those with a narrow spectrum against Gram-positive organisms. Broad-spectrum antibiotics are a little safer, but none are totally free from the risk of inducing this condition. Topical antibiotic preparations will also induce enterotoxaemia if the guinea pig is allowed to lick at them (see Chapter 11 for list of drugs).

Prevention. Where possible the use of antibiotics should be avoided. If they are necessary they are best given subcutaneously or intramuscularly as the oral route carries a lesser safety margin.

If antibiotics must be used they are best given with a probiotic, e.g. live natural yogurt or Vetrumex (Tx 11 or 13), to protect the gut flora.

During a course of antibiotics the uptake of essential vitamins in the gut is also likely to be upset, and administration of vitamin drops concurrently with the antibiotic and in the recovery period is recommended, e.g. Abidec drops (Tx 52).

Colic

This may occur as a sporadic symptom on its own or may accompany a more serious complaint such as gastroenteritis or an abdominal catastrophe, e.g. a torsion.

Clinical signs. The affected animal may appear bloated and will be very tender on abdominal palpation.

Treatment. Non-specific colics will respond well to a kaolin or kaolin and morphine preparation (Tx 23) given 3−4 times daily. If the colic is a symptom of a more serious condition the prognosis is poorer and treatment must be aimed at the cause of the problem.

Intussusception

Clinical signs. This condition has been recorded in a guinea pig after a bout of diarrhoea. The initial scouring appeared to resolve after 5 days and then the guinea pig began to pass small amounts of blood mixed with firm motions. A day later it passed a 10 cm section of gut and the condition resolved completely.

Gastric torsion

This condition is occasionally diagnosed at post-mortem. It causes sudden death which may or may not be preceded by a period of intense abdominal discomfort.

Red droppings

Occasionally the droppings may be well formed but appear to have a dark red coating which may seem like blood. This can usually be related to the feeding of beetroot and should not be a matter for concern. Similarly the urine may also be stained red.

Anorexia

A guinea pig may stop eating for a great variety of reasons and this may be a symptom of many disease conditions. However, it is possible on occasion for an individual to develop a non-specific anorexia in the absence of any other clinical signs.

Treatment. Provided that no other reason for the anorexia can be determined the affected guinea pig can sometimes be stimulated into regaining its appetite by feeding it a mixture of natural yogurt (or other probiotic, e.g. Vetrumex, Tx 13), vitamin C, ground faecal pellets from a healthy cavy and a little soaked dry food. This mixture provides a boost to the normal gastrointestinal flora and is a useful appetite stimulant. An injection of anabolic steroid and multi-B vitamins can also be tried.

6/ The Musculoskeletal System

The feet

The guinea pig has four toes on each foreleg and three toes on each hindleg. Each toe has an associated pad. Each forefoot has a main pad and a pronounced stopper pad. Each hindfoot also has a main pad and a stopper pad which extends along the volar aspect of the metacarpus to the hock joint.

Overgrown toe-nails

The nails of some guinea pigs never need trimming, whilst others require frequent attention, particularly on the front feet where they can grow right round under and into the foot. By the very nature of the soft bedding on which they are kept this problem is fairly common.

Treatment. Regular nail trimming to just below the quick, which is clearly visible if the nails are white. If the quick is accidentally cut the end can be cauterized with a styptic (e.g. potassium permanganate).

If the nail has actually grown into the foot the open wound should be cleansed with a saline solution (Tx 59) and Dermisol cream (Tx 25) or a wound powder applied topically.

Polydactyly

Clinical signs. The presence of an extra toe or toes, usually on the hindlegs. It is sometimes a consequence of close inbreeding.

Treatment. As the extra toes are often only attached by a loose piece of skin breeders may pinch them off between their forefinger and thumb soon after birth. Alternatively they can be removed with a pair of sharp scissors and any subsequent bleeding should be cauterized with potassium permanganate as with dew claw removal in very young puppies.

Bent leg

This condition is occasionally noticed at birth. The front leg is usually affected and this condition is attributed to the position of the fetus in the uterus, although it may be due to a muscle contracture. With careful massage and gentle manipulation the condition may resolve after the first few days of life.

Corns and pressure points

Clinical signs. Corns are a proliferation of horny material between the toes on the underside of the foot. They are most common on the forefeet.

Pressure points have a similar thickening on the point of the hocks and they commonly occur during pregnancy when the hindlegs are carrying more weight than usual.

If the hygiene of the hutch floor is poor, corns will readily become infected and lead to the development of pododermatitis.

Treatment. Any extra horn can be carefully removed with a sharp pair of scissors and the area cleaned with a dilute Pevidine (Tx 57, a povidone-iodine solution). Both corns and pressure points can be softened with a petroleum jelly (Vaseline) or Dermisol cream (Tx 25) which can be rubbed into the affected area twice daily. The hutch floor should be kept clean and any abrasive bedding materials should be avoided.

Pododermatitis

Clinical signs. Swelling and ulceration of the foot pad. In severe cases this may progress to osteoarthritis and amyloidosis of the liver, spleen, kidneys and adrenal glands.

Treatment. The cause of this condition is usually bacterial in origin. The most commonly isolated bacterium is *Staphylococcus aureus*. Treatment of advanced infections where there is marked swelling of the foot is rarely successful. The foot should be cleaned with an antiseptic solution and a topical antibiotic/corticosteroid cream (Tx 28) applied to the affected area. Systemic or parenteral antibiotics (Tx 1–9) should also be administered. If possible the foot should be lightly dressed to prevent any pieces of hay and shavings from aggravating the sore.

An alternative treatment which has been reported to be successful is the injection of antibiotics directly into the affected foot pad. A dose of 0.2 ml lincocin sterile solution (Upjohn Ltd) equivalent to 20 mg lincomycin is injected daily for 5–7 days.

Comment. This condition is generally associated with rough flooring and poor hutch hygiene resulting in feet abrasions which become readily contaminated. By improving the floor surface and with regular hutch cleaning the incidence of this condition should be reduced.

Occasionally similar symptoms are seen as a consequence of a fungal infection, and in these cases treatment with a suitable fungicide can be tried, e.g. Defungit applied as a 0.5% solution every second or third day (Tx 17). Alternatively the foot can be treated with Tinaderm-M cream (Tx 19 containing the anti-fungal agents tolnaftate and nystatin) twice daily.

Paralysis and reluctance to move

Trauma

Guinea pigs are very susceptible to spinal trauma if they are accidently dropped or fall from their hutch.

Clinical signs. These are of acute onset and usually related to the time of a fall. The guinea pig's hindlegs may be totally paralysed and the normal nervous reflexes are usually absent. Urinary incontinence is often an accompanying feature. There may also be a palpable deviation or fracture in the spine and pain around this area. If necessary the diagnosis can be confirmed by radiography.

Treatment. If the damage is severe euthanasia is the kindest option.

Viral

Clinical signs. The affected animal may appear hunched over and unable to raise its head. Other symptoms include pyrexia, or weight loss with gradual muscular weakness and hindleg paralysis.

Treatment. Unsuccessful.

Osteoporosis

This occurs if guinea pigs are over-supplemented with vitamin D, e.g. in the form of cod-liver oil. This leads to calcium resorption from bone and subsequent bone weakness. One of the first clinical signs is paralysis of the hindlegs. If the guinea pig is receiving a balanced diet of dry and green food this supplementation is unnecessary. Sun-dried hay and exposure to sunlight will provide the guinea pig with adequate amounts of this vitamin.

Treatment. The dietary imbalance must be corrected and any vitamin D supplementation must be stopped. It may be helpful to withhold hay for the first few days and give the affected guinea pig extra calcium in the form of Collo-Cal D (Tx 53).

Comment. Vitamin D is often given to enhance the lustre of the coat, but it can be harmful if over-supplementation occurs. It is better to use a combination of polyunsaturated oils, e.g. Vitapet or evening primrose oil, for this purpose.

The diet of the guinea pig must contain the correct ratio of calcium : phosphorus (see metastatic calcification) and no more than 1600 iu of vitamin D per kg.

Metastatic calcification

This condition is also the result of an alteration in the delicate balance of calcium, phosphorus and vitamin D. An imbalance of magnesium and potassium is also involved. However, as commercial diets are now better formulated it is an infrequent problem.

Clinical signs. Metastatic calcification is most often seen in males over a year old and these exhibit joint stiffness, poor weight gain and death.

Pathology. Calcium deposits in skeletal muscle and other organs, especially the stomach, colon, lungs and aorta.

Comment. This condition can be minimized by feeding diets with a calcium : phosphorus ratio of 1.5 : 1 and no more vitamin D than 1600 iu/kg. In practice this can be achieved by a balanced diet of cavy pellets, green foods, carrots and beetroot.

If hyperphosphataemia does occur this leads to a compensatory fall in blood calcium. This hypocalcaemia stimulates the release of parathyroid hormone and calcium is resorbed from bone and deposited in skeletal muscle and many organs in the body, especially in the colon, stomach, aorta and lungs. Hyperphosphataemia occurs when guinea pigs are fed diets low in magnesium and potassium and the condition can be minimized by feeding diets that contain at least 0.35% magnesium.

Rickets

This condition (which is also due to vitamin D deficiency) is extremely rare as a balanced diet provides adequate calcium, phosphorus and vitamin D. Problems may only occur if the guinea pigs are kept in poor light, as sunlight is necessary to stimulate the production of vitamin D in the skin.

Muscular dystrophy

Clinical signs. The affected animal is stiff and reluctant to move.

Pathology. Microscopic lesions include coagulative necrosis, inflammation and proliferation of the sarcolemmal nuclei in skeletal muscle.

Treatment. This condition is due to a vitamin E deficiency. The diet should contain 50 mg of vitamin E per kg. Wheatgerm oil is a useful source of vitamin E.

Scurvy

Clinical signs. Unsteady gait, painful locomotion, haemorrhage from gums, swollen costochondral junctions and poor weight gain or gradual wasting. Sub-clinical scurvy may present as excessive salivation or just a lowering of the guinea pig's resistance to the development of other conditions.

Pathology. Lesions include haemorrhages in the subcutis and in skeletal muscle. Also haemorrhages around the joints (especially the stifle) and on all serosal surfaces. Microscopically there is a disarray of the cartilage columns and fibrosis in areas of active osteogenesis.

Treatment. An affected animal must be given 50–100 mg vitamin C per day, preferably as drops given orally until the condition resolves.

Comment. The condition is due to a deficiency of vitamin C (ascorbic acid). An adult guinea pig requires 10–30 mg of vitamin C per day. Supplementation can be achieved by dissolving soluble vitamin C tablets (Tx 54) in the drinking water (average water consumption is 8 ml per 100 g bodyweight) or by provision of adequate greenstuffs. Beetroot and carrots contain 3 mg per 25 g of vitamin C, and cabbage and spinach contain 17–20 mg per 25 g. Most proprietory guinea pig pellets contain adequate amounts of this vitamin provided that they have not been stored for longer than 3 months. Rabbit pellets, however, may contain little or no vitamin C.

Guinea pigs lack the enzymes necessary to convert L-gulonolactone to L-ascorbic acid and therefore require a dietary supplement of ascorbic acid. The normal requirement is 10 mg per kg body weight and this increases twofold during pregnancy.

There is no risk of over-supplementation with this vitamin as any excess is excreted through the kidneys.

Systemic disease

Infections with bacteria such as *Bordetella* and *Streptococcus* spp. will also produce a hunched-up posture and the affected individual will be disinclined to move.

Fractures

Limb fractures are usually sustained as a result of a fall as a consequence of the guinea pig being dropped. Rib fractures and subsequent chest injury are commonly seen in guinea pigs housed with rabbits. These fractures are usually the result of a kick from the rabbit's powerful hindlegs.

Treatment. Limb fractures will respond well to external fixation providing that they are adequately immobilized. External support is usually required for 3–4 weeks. Even if the limb is not returned to its full function the guinea pig will be able to cope adequately.

Osteomyelitis

Clinical signs. Lameness and swelling of one or more joints.

Treatment. Broad-spectrum antibiotics (Tx 1−9).

Comment. The most common bacterial agents are *Staphylococcus aureus*, *Streptococcus monoiliformis*, *Pasturella multocida* and other streptococcal species. This condition may be a sequel to pododermatitis as the likely route of infection is via an abrasion on the foot. Prevention must include improving the standard of the hutch hygiene and removal of any abrasive flooring.

7/ The Head and Neck

7.1 The eye

Microphthalmia

Clinical signs. The eye is small or non-existent and the guinea pig is therefore blind. This condition is generally associated with all white-coated guinea pigs which are a result of either a Dalmation × Dalmation or a roan × roan mating. The offspring are known as 'microphthalmic whites'. Both these breeds should only be mated with self-colours, or self-coloured carriers.

Comment. The gene producing the roan coat colour is associated with a lethal gene which produces abnormalities of the eyes and occasionally accompanying disorders of the digestive tract.

Foreign bodies

Hay seeds commonly find their way into the eyes of guinea pigs. If undetected they may cause corneal ulceration and corneal oedema.

Clinical signs. Blepharospasm, epiphora and ocular discharge. Often unilateral conjunctivitis.

Treatment. A drop of local anaesthetic (Ophthaine) can be placed in the eye and it should then be possible to remove the seed with forceps, or with a piece of damp cotton wool. If there has been no corneal damage, a topical antibiotic/steroid ointment (e.g. Chloromycetin hydrocortisone or Neobiotic HC drops, Tx 31–33) can be used for the following few days. If corneal ulceration is present, a topical antibiotic preparation should be used alone (e.g. Cepravin Tx 30). However, in cases accompanied by severe conjunctivitis Panalog is very effective in the acute stages. Application of all preparations should be made frequently (four times daily if possible).

Corneal ulceration

This is a common sequel to a foreign body in the eye or it may be the result of damage to the cornea by a sharp piece of straw. Corneal damage is evident and corneal oedema is generally present. If healing has begun, blood vessels will be seen running towards the ulcer from the scleral margin.

Corneal oedema may be seen in one-day-old guinea pigs caused unintentionally by their mother whilst cleaning them. However, it can also be due to entropion (see below).

Treatment. Topical application of an antibiotic eye preparation twice daily, e.g. Cepravin (Tx 30) or Orbenin eye preparations. If necessary the eye can be bathed with a dilute saline solution (Tx 59). If the ulcer is not severe it will heal in 7−10 days (see also treatment of foreign bodies above).

Conjunctivitis

Clinical signs. The conjunctiva are reddened and there may be epiphora or an ocular discharge. It is seen as a symptom of upper respiratory disease, as an allergic response, or secondary to irritation and local trauma. In the latter case the condition is usually unilateral, whilst bilateral conjunctivitis is usually a symptom of a more generalized condition.

A transient conjunctivitis associated with *Candida albicans* has also been recorded.

Treatment. If there is no corneal damage topical applications of an antibiotic/steroid preparation (Tx 31−33) should be given 3−4 times daily. .

If it appears to be a summer (pollen) allergy, Betsolan eye drops (Tx 34) will be effective. A mild saline solution (a teaspoon of salt to a pint of water) applied to the eye by a dropper three times daily will also bring some relief to the affected individual. In allergy cases the swelling of the conjunctiva may also be accompanied by swelling of the eyelids.

Chlamydial neonatal conjunctivitis

Clinical signs. A bilateral conjunctivitis which is present at, or soon after, birth. There may be marked inflammation and chemosis.

Treatment. A topical antibiotic/steroid eye preparation (Tx 31–33) will resolve this condition. However, the condition is self-limiting and may resolve without treatment.

Entropion

Clinical signs. In-turning of the eyelid causing the eyelashes to rub against the cornea. This condition generally affects the lower eyelid and may be unilateral or bilateral. Affected youngsters will be born with corneal oedema or this may develop in the first few days of life. Minute areas of corneal ulceration may be visible.

Treatment. Often no treatment is required although topical application of a suitable antibiotic eye preparation (Tx 29–30) will relieve the condition until the entropion corrects itself.

Comment. This condition is especially prevalent in the Texel breed. The corneal oedema will resolve after treatment and there is no permanent damage to the eye. The corneal damage occurs *in utero* whilst the eyes are shut, but since guinea pigs are born with their eyes open the eyelashes do not usually interfere with the cornea after birth. Most entropions which are present at birth correct themselves within the first 14 days of life.

Congenital cataracts

Cataracts which are present at birth have been seen in some lines of Abyssinians, and breeders may refer to this condition as 'mirror eye'. Related individuals may develop similar cataracts in early adulthood. The mode of inheritance is unknown although studies suggest it may be sex-linked. None of the progeny from such an affected line should be used for further breeding.

Some youngsters may be born with partial cataracts which do not appear to progress as the guinea pig ages, and these small cataracts do not usually compromise vision.

Cataracts

Cases have been recorded where cataracts have developed when the guinea pig is 9–10 months old and the condition is often unilateral. This is an inherited condition although the mode of inheritance is unclear. It is advisable to remove the affected guinea pig and its progeny from the breeding programme as soon as the condition is diagnosed otherwise it will reappear in future generations.

The author has also seen bilateral cataracts develop in a group of related guinea pigs at the age of 2–3 years. This condition also seems to be inherited and as only sows are affected it is therefore suggested that the mode of inheritance may be sex-linked.

In cases of both unilateral or bilateral cataracts the guinea pig is often able to cope adequately relying on its senses of smell and hearing especially if it is kept in familiar surroundings. In the early stages the pupillary light reflex is often still present, suggesting that the affected individuals may retain some degree of sight.

Lens luxation

Bilateral lens luxation has been seen in an Abyssinian secondary to cataract formation.

On ophthalmic examination, an aphakic crescent is visible between the lens equator and the iris.

Adequate vision will be present unless the eye develops secondary glaucoma.

Milky ocular discharge

The presence of this discharge is often a cause for concern, but it is a normal fluid which is released from the eye as part of the grooming process. However, it must be differentiated from ocular discharges that accompany pathological changes in the eye.

'Fatty eye'

This is a term used to describe a permanent protrusion of the lower conjunctival sac. This condition is most common in Self-Whites, Blacks and Creams and also Rexes. It is thought to be an inherited condition.

'Red eye'

This is a term used to describe a similar protrusion of the lower conjunctival sac. However, in contrast to 'fatty eye' this condition is not present all the time but appears at times of stress or when the eye is exposed to irritant substances such as cigarette smoke.

Treatment. Betsolan eye drops (Tx 34) will reduce the inflammation.

7.2   The ear

Anatomy

The internal structure of the ear is essentially similar to that of all other mammals, however, the cochlea of the guinea pig has four coils, and they therefore possess very acute hearing. In comparison with the majority of other rodents the guinea pig has very large tympanic bullae.

Aural haematoma

Clinical signs. The pinna is swollen and feels full of fluid. It may be slightly warmer than normal. This condition must be differentiated from an abscess.

Treatment. This condition does not usually bother the affected guinea pig and it is probably best left alone to clot and shrink naturally by the process of clot resorption and fibrosis. However, if the guinea pig is a show animal an attempt can be made to drain the haematoma and reduce the swelling by suturing the ear between two buttons which will keep the pinna under constant pressure. The affected individual must be isolated otherwise its companions are likely to chew at the sutures. The sutures should be left in for at least 2 weeks.

Wounds

These are usually a result of fighting. Tears and lacerations are common injuries which may be obtained during disputes over feeding bowls. Young guinea pigs may receive ear injuries if their mother is startled whilst she is feeding them and she accidentally catches their ears with her nails as she moves.

Treatment. If the wound is still bleeding digital pressure should be applied. The ear should be held between finger and thumb for at least 5 minutes. If this is ineffective a small piece of Granuflex can be sutured over the wound. This will act as a pressure pad and also aid subsequent healing.

Older wounds can be bathed in a dilute salt solution (Tx 59) and dusted with an antiseptic wound powder.

Comment. Adequate numbers of feeding bowls must be provided to avoid head-to-head disputes over food.

Solar dermatitis

Clinical signs. This condition usually affects white guinea pigs with pink ears and occurs when they are exposed to sunlight. The pinnae become hot and inflamed.

Treatment. The affected guinea pig must be removed from the direct sunlight and the ears can be treated with a topical steroid cream (Tx 28).

Prevention. Affected cavies should not be exposed to too much direct sunlight. Their ears can be protected by using an infant sun-blocking preparation.

Middle ear disease

Clinical signs. The guinea pig holds its head over to the affected side and may fall over to the same side, due to a disturbance of its sense of balance.

Diagnosis. Pus may be seen in the ear canal. However, radiography of the tympanic bullae is often more useful than otoscopy as the changes in these large bullae are usually severe. Radiography will reveal a marked thickening of the bone of the tympanic bullae diagnostic of otitis media and this may be present in the absence of a purulent discharge.

Treatment. This is generally unrewarding as antibiotics, either parenteral or intra-aural, fail to reach the centre of the infection. If the guinea pig is otherwise well and is a single pet it is better left and allowed to compensate for its altered posture. Guinea pigs that are part of a large breeding unit are better destroyed to avoid the risk of the spread of infection.

Comment. This condition must be differentiated from wry neck, a congenital problem which causes a deformity in newborn guinea pigs, and which will also cause the guinea pig to hold its head over to one side (see section 7.4). Middle ear disease may progress to affect the inner ear and subsequently the adjacent part of the meninges and brain. In these cases the clinical signs of circling, falling to the affected side and torticollis will persist.

This syndrome is often a sequel to a prurulent upper respiratory tract infection associated commonly with *Streptococcus* and *Pasturella* spp. However, it may also accompany respiratory tract infections yet remain clinically inapparent. Otitis media is a common finding at post-mortem in individuals which have never exhibited clinical signs associated with this condition.

7.3   The mouth

The teeth

Anatomy

The guinea pig has two upper and two lower incisors for gnawing. These teeth only have enamel on their front surfaces and are therefore self-sharpening. The canines are absent but in their place is a gap known as the diastema. There are four upper and lower cheek teeth (one premolar and three molars) on both sides. Guinea pigs' teeth are open-rooted and grow continuously (hyspiodontic) and therefore they must be provided with a constant supply of hard food to ensure even wearing of the teeth.

Congenital absence of teeth. On rare occasions young are born without any teeth, and although they appear normal for the first 24 hours they then take on a starved hunched appearance as they cannot eat. They should be culled as they will not grow teeth later. As this is a genetic fault the parents of these affected young should not be bred from again.

Broken teeth

These commonly occur as a result of falls or fighting.

Treatment. The teeth must be clipped level to provide an even bite surface. It is doubly important that the guinea pig is supplied with hard foods at this time to keep the teeth even, as the feeding of soft foods will lead to uncontrolled growth of the other teeth.

Weak teeth

Clinical signs. The teeth break very easily, or may drop out if knocked.

Treatment. This can be a sign of vitamin D deficiency. Lack of this vitamin leads to a calcium deficiency and therefore poorly mineralized teeth and bones. The cavy acquires its vitamin D from two sources — from its diet and from the synthesis of vitamin D via its skin in daylight. It is only when it is deprived of both sources that teeth and bone weaknesses occur.

Excess vitamin D is harmful but in severely affected cases one drop of cod-liver oil can be given orally for a week. At the same time the diet must be improved and the sunlight to the caviary increased. Alternatively a calcium and vitamin D supplement can be given (Tx 53).

Wasting disease

Clinical signs. The guinea pig loses weight, especially from the hindquarters. It also gradually becomes anorexic and usually salivates profusely.

Treatment. These signs are often attributable to overgrowth of the molars, even to the extent that they impinge on the cheek or tongue. The hard ridges of the molars can sometimes be felt by external palpation through the cheeks. A special gag is needed if these teeth are to be clipped and filed, and the procedure often requires a general anaesthetic. However, an elastrator ring expander may provide a cheap alternative to specialist equipment. The prognosis for these cases is poor, as even once the teeth are clipped they are likely to regrow again quite quickly.

Comment. 'Wasting disease' may sometimes be due to a vitamin C deficiency, and recently diabetes mellitus has been implicated as a cause. It is very important to differentiate between these conditions so that the proper treatment can be given.

Malocclusions

An undershot jaw presentation is fairly common and this leads to the improper wear of the front incisors which will need regular clipping.

Malocclusion of the cheek teeth (see wasting disease above) is an inherited condition and affected individuals and their offspring should not be bred from.

Tooth root abscesses

Clinical signs. The guinea pig stops eating and may salivate profusely. Occasionally pus may be seen coming from the back of the mouth. The molars are usually affected by this condition and they can be examined satisfactorily by using an aural speculum (preferably metal).

Treatment. Broad-spectrum antibiotics (Tx 1–9) can be tried but usually once the condition is detected the guinea pig is unlikely to respond and start eating again. A special mouth gag is required if the tooth is to be removed under general anaesthesia, as the anatomy of the mouth with the abundance of loose buccal skin does not lend itself easily to this kind of procedure.

Cleft palate

This congenital abnormality is obvious a few days after birth. The affected guinea pig is unable to suckle properly and food may be seen running down the nose. The cleft usually involves the hard palate only, and may vary from a small defect to the severe case which runs the whole length of the hard palate. There is no treatment for this and the guinea pig should be destroyed. As the condition is inherited the parents of the affected individual should not be bred from again.

Ptyalism (slobbers)

Slobbering can occur as a result of overgrown teeth, as a symptom of heatstroke and it is also seen in cases of hypovitaminosis C. Salivation may also be a clinical sign of ketosis.

The lips

Scabs around the mouth: mild form

Clinical signs. The guinea pig has multiple scabs especially in the corners of the lips. If the condition is severe these can spread up over the nose. The affected animal is usually still in good health and eating normally.

Treatment. Cleanse the scabs around the mouth with an antiseptic solution daily. A dilute solution of Pevidine (povidone-iodine, Tx 57) is recommended. Panalog ointment or cream (Tx 27) should then be applied twice daily to the affected area. Alternatively the sores can be painted with gentian violet. The latter is the preferred method of treatment if the affected cavy is pregnant as antibiotics are best avoided during gestation.

Scabs around the mouth: severe form

Clinical signs. The scabs may progress to include the gums and in turn the teeth may become brittle. Septicaemia and death are common.

Treatment. This condition is incurable and euthanasia should be considered.

Comment. Both forms are contagious and are spread via infected food dishes and drinkers and wire doors.

The milder form is more common. It is wise to isolate the

affected guinea pig once the condition is diagnosed and the treatment should be successful, although there may be a recurrence of the condition at a later date.

The bacteria usually gain entry via small abrasions at the edges of the mouth from sharp pieces of food or from constant chewing by the guinea pig at its bars. It is wise to remove all abrasive foodstuffs to minimize the occurrence of this problem. All food bowls and drinkers should be sterilized and the wire fronts of the hutch doors scrubbed with an antiseptic (e.g. dilute Savlon solution Tx 58).

The eating of foods with a high acid content may predispose the guinea pig to the development of this condition and beetroot and apples should be removed from the affected individual's diet.

Sialitis

Clinical signs. Swelling of the throat in the region of the salivary glands and excess salivation.

Pathology. The formation of large eosinophilic intranuclear inclusion bodies in the epithelium of the salivary duct.

Comment. This may be due to a viral infection (cytomegalovirus). There is no treatment, but the condition may resolve with supportive therapy. Often the infection may be asymptomatic.

7.4   The neck

Cervical lymphadenitis

Clinical signs. Large, often unilateral swellings or abscesses in the ventral region of the neck. These swellings are in the cervical lymph nodes and are usually caused by an infection with *Streptococcus zooepidemicus* although other bacteria can cause the same condition. In some cases death may occur as a result of septicaemia.

Treatment. Fourteen days of daily administration of 25 mg/kg cephaloridine (Tx 1, Ceporin, Coopers Pitman-Moore) intramuscularly should control and eliminate the condition. However, Ceporin has now largely been replaced by cephalexin (Tx 2, Ceporex, Coopers Pitman-Moore) the dose of which is 50–100 mg/kg intramuscularly.

Comment. The causal organism usually gains access to the lymph nodes via abrasions of the oral mucosa or via the upper respiratory tract. Thus the use of abrasive materials in the feed or bedding should be avoided. As the material from discharging abscesses is highly contagious the affected animal should be isolated for treatment. If the animal is part of a large breeding colony it may be advisable to cull it to prevent the disease becoming enzootic.

Other bacteria which are frequently isolated are *Streptococcus monoiliformis*, *Fusiformis* and *Pasturella* spp.

Foreign bodies

Clinical signs. A swelling in the throat region which is not associated with a lymph node. It may be hot and painful on palpation.

Comment. These abscesses are usually the result of a thistle from the hay which penetrates through the mucous membranes of the mouth and tracks under the chin.

Treatment. If the abscess bursts it can be bathed with a saline solution and the flushed with 3% hydrogen peroxide (Tx 56). A topical preparation such as Dermisol (Tx 25) can then be used to assist healing.

If the abscess has not burst it can be brought to a head by the use of warm poultices, and then treated as above.

If the position or size of the abscess is such that it compromises swallowing or causes great discomfort to the guinea pig it should be lanced and drained. It may be necessary to administer a general anaesthetic for this procedure.

Wry neck

This condition is seen in newborn guinea pigs. The severity of the condition is variable. The young exhibit degrees of torticollis, and those which are very badly affected may have to lie on their backs to suckle due to their abnormal head posture. More mildly affected individuals with only a slight deformity will be able to compensate and will appear near normal after 2–3 days.

This condition is hereditary and the parents of affected offspring should not be used for breeding again.

The thymus

In young guinea pigs this organ is present and palpable subcutaneously on either side of the trachea and within the neck. This is
a clinically normal finding and should not be mistaken for a pathological condition.

8/ Behaviour and the Central Nervous System

Aggression

This is usually only a problem if boars are housed together. It is best to pen adult boars separately or with other females. Two young boars from the same litter may live in harmony if there are no females present. However, as they reach adulthood one will begin to exert its dominance and they may start fighting.

There is often an initial show of aggression when guinea pigs are penned together for the first time, but this will generally only be temporary, and will settle down once the 'pecking order' has been established. The aggressive animal will adopt a defensive posture and chatter its teeth in warning. The hair on its neck and shoulders may stand erect. These conflicts should not last longer than 2−3 hours and if they do it is better to separate the offenders.

One procedure that can be tried to minimize this problem is to smear a little mentholated vapour rub (e.g. Vick) around the rump and under the chin of the original guinea pigs and of the newcomers. This eliminates the differences in the body odours of the two groups and often removes the trigger for conflict. It is also advisable to mix the two groups in mutual surroundings so that territory-protecting is not a component of any disagreements.

Unfortunately some sows may become aggressive when housed with other sows. Often the introduction of a boar will quieten an aggressive sow, or if necessary, she can be removed from the pen and housed separately with a boar.

It is important to provide plenty of food, and if necessary two or more bowls of dry mix in order to keep any disputes over feeding space to a minimum.

Epilepsy

Clinical signs. The affected guinea pig has a classic epileptic fit which can last for anything up to 3−4 minutes during which time it salivates profusely and lies on its side twitching its limbs. There then follows a post-ictal period when it may exhibit abnormal behaviour such as polyphagia and aggression.

Treatment. Often as the frequency of the fits increases the affected animals are euthanased. The use of an anti-convulsant such as primidone (Tx 49, Mysoline) is a suggested alternative.

Fits

Guinea pigs may also have fits which are not true epileptiform convulsions. The fits may take the form of mild twitching or full seizures. They are usually secondary to another disease process and the prognosis is poor. Euthanasia is often the necessary outcome.

Fits such as these occur as a result of liver and kidney failure, ketosis, enterotoxaemia and septicaemia. They may also occur in cavies with severe mycosis.

Convulsions may also be seen in guinea pigs which are very badly affected with severe pruritus caused by *Trixacarus caviae*, the mange mite. If the mange is treated successfully the fits will cease. Whilst ectoparasitic treatment is in progress any seizures can be controlled with diazepam (Tx 51) given by intramuscular injection at a dose of 1–2 mg/kg. Affected guinea pigs can then be maintained on primidone (Tx 49, Mysoline suspension).

Neonatal neurological deficits

Varying degrees of brain damage may be seen in youngsters which have suffered the trauma of a lengthy and difficult birth. These youngsters are often very uncoordinated and are unable to suckle properly. Hand-rearing is unsatisfactory as the affected young are unable to compensate for their disabilities, and euthanasia should be the considered option.

Fetuses which suffer central nervous defects of a genetic nature are usually aborted, or are stillborn at birth.

Cerebellar disease

Clinical signs. Torticollis. The guinea pig may circle to one side, and may also fall over to the same side. Nystagmus seems to be a very infrequent clinical sign in affected guinea pigs.

Comment. These signs are almost always secondary to a middle ear infection which has progressed to the inner ear and the meninges. Encephalopathies leading to torticollis are very rare.

Similar symptoms have been seen following a CVA (cerebral vascular accident). Whatever the initiating cause of these symptoms the prognosis is poor.

Treatment. If a CVA is suspected an injection of steroids (e.g. betamethasone, Tx 44) can be given. Treatment of middle ear disease with antibiotics is usually unrewarding, and if the guinea pig is part of a large breeding unit it is best to consider euthanasia as it is a potential source of infection for others.

9/ Husbandry

Introduction

There is a wealth of literature which is already available on this subject. The aims of this chapter are to discuss guinea pig management in relation to the prevention and treatment of disease conditions.

9.1 Housing

The commonest method of housing guinea pigs is in a hutch. However, they can be kept in a wide range of cage types, from converted cupboards to large cardboard boxes! Some guinea pigs are housed in wire cages with mesh floors.

Outdoor hutches can be covered with roofing felt, or a similar material, which will provide protection against bad weather. They should not be treated with creosote, as this is toxic to guinea pigs and will cause severe liver damage if the fumes are inhaled.

Size of accommodation

Each guinea pig should be allowed a minimum floor area of 0.2 m². The cages should be at least 25 cm high.

However, a larger area for exercise is beneficial, and this can be provided either in the form of indoor floor runs, or as outdoor grass runs. The latter should be covered with mesh or netting to protect the guinea pigs from cats and other predators. The provision of adequate exercise is especially important for sows during pregnancy as it may help prevent the development of pregnancy toxaemia.

The flooring

If wire floors are used care must be taken to ensure that there are no abrasive surfaces which could cause foot damage and subsequent pododermatitis. A mesh of 1.25 × 3.5 cm or smaller will prevent the guinea pigs trapping their feet in the wire holes.

The preferred bedding material is a layer of newspaper which is covered with woodshavings and hay. If woodshavings are used it is important that they are made only from untreated soft woods, as certain hard woods have toxic properties. Sawdust is not recommended for use as a bedding material as it is too fine and particles may easily become lodged in the guinea pig's eye if it tries to burrow under the bedding. Sawdust has also been found lodged in the prepuce of males causing impaction and infection.

Straw is also not recommended as it is abrasive by nature, and is responsible for causing a large proportion of eye injuries.

Hygiene

The accommodation should be cleaned out regularly. If the litter is allowed to build up there will be an accumulation of ammonia and this weakens the resistance of the respiratory tract to infection.

As the guinea pig's urine often contains small crystals of ammonium phosphate and calcium carbonate there may be a build up of scale around the hutch. This can be removed by cleaning with a weak acid solution (e.g. dilute acetic acid).

Environment

The guinea pigs should be kept away from draughts and protected against extremes of temperature. They should receive adequate amounts of light, but should not be exposed to direct sunlight during the summer as they are very susceptible to the development of heatstroke (see below). Recommendations for the environmental temperature and humidity are:
- Temperature: 20–22°C (68–72°F).
- Humidity: 45–65%.

These figures apply for optimum performance, however, guinea pigs can be quite safely kept at much lower temperatures (such as those we experience during our British winters) providing that they are protected from draughts. At temperatures above 29°C there is a high incidence of infertility problems and early abortions.

Heatstroke

Guinea pigs are prone to developing heat stroke when exposed
to high environmental temperatures (above 28°C) or when kept
in grass runs exposed to strong sunlight. Heavily pregnant females
are the most susceptible, and the problem is worse if they are
deprived of water at the same time. They are also particularly
susceptible during car journeys to shows, and at shows too, if
their show pen is in direct sunlight.

Clinical signs. Rapid respiration, salivation, prostration and
eventually death.

Treatment. They must be cooled rapidly. If necessary their body
can be immersed in cold water. An injection of steroids (e.g.
betamethasone Tx 44) may be beneficial.

9.2   Nutrition

Many disease conditions in guinea pigs can be related to the feeding
of an incorrect diet. It is very important to provide a well-balanced
diet and the following sections aim to discuss a few basic principles
of guinea pig nutrition and describe the qualities of common foodstuffs and their relationship to disease conditions.

Principles of guinea pig nutrition

1   The guinea pig, like humans and apes, is unable to synthesize
its own vitamin C (ascorbic acid) as it lacks the enzyme L-
gulonolactone oxidase which is required to convert L-gulonolactone to L-ascorbic acid. It therefore requires a daily supply of
vitamin C. The normal requirement for vitamin C is 10 mg/kg,
and this increases to 20 mg/kg during pregnancy.

   If vitamin C is added to the drinking water in the form of
soluble tablets (Tx 54) it must be given via a dish or a bottle
with a stainless steel nozzle. Other metals will accelerate the
decomposition of ascorbic acid. Rosehip syrup is a useful
alternative which can be added to the drinking water to provide
extra vitamin C. It should be diluted with water to produce a
solution containing 12 mg per 100 ml of vitamin C.

The daily requirements for this vitamin will be met as long as a balanced diet of dry food, carrots and greens is fed. The vitamin C content of dried food will deteriorate over 9−12 weeks, so deficiency problems will arise if the dry food is stale. Rabbit food is also unsuitable as it does not contain adequate amounts of this vitamin.

Hypervitaminosis C is not a recognized problem as any ascorbic acid which is excess to requirements is excreted through the kidneys.

2 Any dietary change must be made slowly, e.g. the introduction of grass and hedgerow plants once their supply becomes plentiful in the spring. Sudden changes will cause diarrhoea and digestive disturbances.

3 A balanced diet must include the following every day:
- Concentrates — the dry food.
- Roots — carrots or beetroot.
- Green foods — cultivated or hedgerow plants.
- Hay — of good quality.
- Fresh water.

If this balance of diet is adhered to there should be little need for extra supplementation, except in a few special cases. Over-zealous vitamin and mineral supplementation may actually unbalance the diet and cause disease problems, e.g. vitamin D overdose if cod-liver oil is added to the diet.

Most of the required vitamins are actually synthesized by the intestinal flora.

4 All food should be fed fresh with no mould on it. Any dry food and greenstuffs which have not been eaten after a few hours should be removed and not allowed to rot in the hutch as this will lead to digestive upsets.

5 Frosted food must not be fed as it will cause digestive upsets. Food should be allowed to thaw if it is kept in the refrigerator, and any fresh food remaining in the hutch should be removed at night during the cold winters as it is likely to freeze overnight.

6 The diet of a young guinea pig should be as varied as possible. It is at this age that the guinea pig is learning about foodstuffs and what it will eat as an adult reflects what it was fed as a youngster. If a guinea pig is offered a new food as an adult it is unlikely to accept it unless it starts to copy other adults in the pen which may be eating it.

7 As the guinea pig is always eating, a supply of hay must be constantly available to prevent boredom. Guinea pigs which have plenty of hay to eat are less likely to develop vices like hair chewing.

Deficiency diseases

Scurvy

This is the result of a vitamin C deficiency. Sub-clinical deficiency lowers the guinea pig's resistance and predisposes it to the development of bacterial pneumonia, acute enteritis, and skin conditions, especially ringworm.

Clinical signs. General unthriftiness, poor weight gain and gradual wasting. Also reluctance to move and lameness. Less commonly seen are haemorrhages from the gums. Excess salivation may be seen in sub-clinical cases.

Pathology. Haemorrhages in the subcutis and in skeletal muscle. Haemorrhages around the joints, especially the stifle, and on all serosal surfaces. Microscopically there is disarray of the cartilage columns and fibrosis in areas of active osteogenesis.

Treatment. Affected cases should be given 50–100 mg/kg vitamin C a day preferably as drops until the condition resolves.

Comment. See notes on vitamin C at the beginning of the nutrition section.

Muscular dystrophy

This is due to an alpha-tocopherol (vitamin E) deficiency. Guinea pigs are particularly sensitive to this deficiency. However, if the guinea pig is receiving a properly balanced commercial diet this deficiency is unlikely to arise.

Clinical signs. Stiffness and reluctance to move.

Pathology. A coagulative necrosis, and inflammation and proliferation of the sarcolemmal nuclei in skeletal muscle.

Treatment. Adequate provision of vitamin E. The diet should contain 50 mg/kg of feed. Affected individuals can be given wheatgerm oil as a liquid form of vitamin E.

Comment. A diet lacking in vitamin E may also lead to infertility problems.

Metastatic calcification

This condition is secondary to an alteration in the complex relationship between calcium, phosphorus, magnesium and potassium. However, as commercial diets are now better formulated this is an infrequent problem.

Clinical signs. This condition is seen most commonly in boars over a year of age. Soft tissue deposits of calcium may lead to lameness, joint stiffness, unthriftiness and death or they may just be an incidental finding at post-mortem examination.

Pathology. Calcium deposits are found in the colon, stomach, aorta and lungs. Many other organs may also be affected.

Comment. This condition can be minimized by feeding diets with a calcium:potassium ratio of 1.5:1 and no more vitamin D than 1600 iu/kg. In practice this can be achieved by feeding a balanced diet of good hay, dry food, greens, carrots and beetroot.

Atrophy or 'wasting disease'

Clinical signs. This condition is characterized by weight loss, especially of the hindlegs and flanks, which may progress to paralysis, a scurfy coat, and salivation. The affected guinea pig continues to eat well despite the progression of the disease.

Comment. The aetiology of this condition is unclear. It is often considered to be due to a vitamin deficiency, particularly of vitamin C. Overgrown teeth have also been implicated as the cause. However, some affected guinea pigs have no teeth problems and are fed a balanced diet. Recently diabetes mellitus has been suggested as a possible cause.

Treatment. The molars can be checked using an aural speculum and if they are overgrown they can be clipped. However, the problem is likely to recur as they will continue to grow (see Chapter 7).

If the diet is inadequate it must be improved. Vitamin C can be given at 100 mg per day until the condition resolves.

One reported case resolved with a good diet and intensive nursing which included daily warm baths and hindleg massage.

Unfortunately not all cases recover and in the case of severely affected cavies euthanasia should be considered.

Vitamin K deficiency

Clinical signs. Epistaxis, intra-uterine haemorrhage, post-partum haemorrhage seen especially in guinea pigs fed only on poor hay and stale dry food.

Treatment. An injection of vitamin K can be given intramuscularly (Konakion, Roche) at a dose of 0.5−1 mg/kg. Vitamin K can then be given orally, and the diet should be improved.

Comment. The recommended requirement of this vitamin is 2 mg/ kg of feed.

Food values of cultivated crops

Beetroot. Contains folic acid, calcium, iron, sodium and vitamin C (3 mg per 28 g), also vitamins B_1 and B_2. Too many leafy tops must not be fed as they contain high levels of oxalic acid which will cause acute renal failure.

Broccoli. Contains vitamins A and B_2, folic acid and vitamin C (17−20 mg per 28 g). Both white and purple sprouting varieties can be fed.

Brussel sprouts. The leaves of these plants can be given. They contain vitamin C (17−20 mg per 28 g) and also vitamins A and B_6, and folic acid.

Cabbage. Contains vitamins A and B_6, folic acid and vitamin C (17−20 mg per 28 g). It also contains calcium, iron, copper and potassium. Cavies will eat green and spring cabbage, but will not always touch the harder white cabbage.

Carrot. Contains calcium, iron, sodium and vitamins A, B_1, B_2, B_6 and C (3 mg per 28 g). The carrot tops are also enjoyed.

Celery. Contains 2 mg per 28 g of vitamin C, and also vitamins A and B_1. The leaves and stalks can both be fed.

Cauliflower. The outside leaves can be given and their food value is approximately the same as cabbage.

Lettuce. Should only be fed in small amounts. It contains 3 mg per 28 g of vitamin C, but it also contains the substance laudanum, which can be harmful.

Spinach. This contains calcium, iron, sodium, potassium and magnesium. It also contains vitamins A, B_2, B_6, E and C, and folic acid ($17-20$ mg/kg).

Swede. This contains 7 mg per 28 g of vitamin C but its quality rapidly deteriorates during storing and it readily goes dry and fibrous.

Watercress. This can be fed as a treat. It contains calcium and sodium and vitamins A and C, and folic acid.

Food values of fruit

Apple. Contains 1 mg per 28 g of vitamin C. They can be fed as a treat, but not given in large quantities as they are fairly acidic.

Wild plants

Plants collected from the hedgerows provide a varied and interesting diet. They must be:
1 Collected away from areas soiled by dogs.
2 Free from bird droppings.
3 Not from areas where weedkiller or pesticide has been used.
4 Not from roadsides close to car exhaust fumes.
See Table 9.1 for a list of poisonous plants which must be avoided.

Table 9.1 Poisonous plants. These include *all* plants that grow from bulbs

Bracken	Horsetails
Bryony	Lily of the valley
Buttercup (this is safe if fed dried in hay)	Mayweeds
Charlock	Monkshood
Convolvulus (bindweed)	Privet
Deadly nightshade	Ragwort
Foxglove	Speedwell
Hellebore	Toadflax
Hemlock	Wild celery
Henbane	

The main principle of feeding hedgerow plants is to provide the guinea pig with a balance of plants with laxative and those with astringent properties. If too many with a laxative effect are fed diarrhoea will occur, and conversely excess astringents may lead to constipation. However, these properties can be used beneficially to correct digestive disturbances and the feeding of astringents only may resolve a case of diarrhoea of dietary origin.

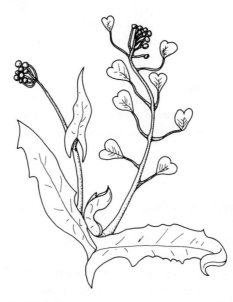

Fig. 9.1 Shepherd's purse.

Astringents

1 Bramble leaves (with the thorns removed).
2 Shepherd's purse (see Fig. 9.1).
3 Docks. These must only be fed before the flower stalks appear. After this their content of oxalic acid rises and too many will cause renal failure.
4 Cleavers (goosegrass) (see Fig. 9.2).

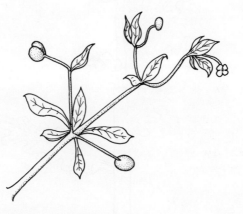

Fig. 9.2 Cleavers (goosegrass).

Laxatives

1 Dandelions.
2 Groundsel (see Fig. 9.3).

Other plants

1 Grass is a very valuable food during the summer and the guinea pig can live in a grass run all day. Care must be taken if feeding grass clippings as they overheat very quickly and cause diarrhoea.
2 Milk thistle (sow thistle). Useful for lactating sows.
3 Vetches.
4 Yarrow (see Fig. 9.4).
5 Coltsfoot. This was used as an old remedy for treating colds and asthma.

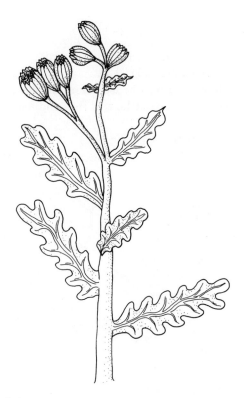

Fig. 9.3 Groundsel.

Dry food

In this category are pellets and cereals (bran, oats, barley and flaked maize). The pellets should contain adequate quantities of vitamin C, although this will deteriorate if they are stored for over 6 weeks. Excess rabbit pellets may cause 'broken back' (see Chapter 1). This condition may also occur if too much flaked maize or barley is included in the diet as both of these foods have overheating properties.

As all foodstuffs in this category are of high calorific value they must not be fed in large quantities to pregnant sows as an obese sow is more prone to developing pregnancy toxaemia or dystocia. The practice of feeding molasses-enriched mixes must be considered carefully because these too are high in calories.

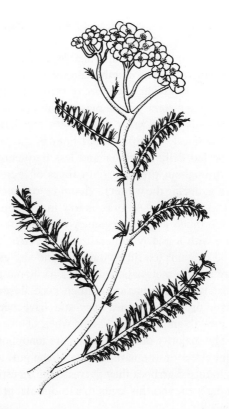

Fig. 9.4 Yarrow.

The nutritional requirements of the guinea pig are as follows:

1 For maintenance:
  - Oil — 2.6%.
  - Protein — 13%.
  - Fibre — 8%.
  - Ash — 6.5%.

2 For breeding:
  - Oil — 3.5%.
  - Protein — 18%.
  - Fibre — 11.2%.
  - Ash — 7.3%.

Some dry mixes sold for small animals in pet shops do approximate quite closely to these requirements. The protein content is the most important factor as diets too low in protein will lead to retarded growth and reduced breeding capacity, whereas diets too high in protein (over 22%) may lead to an increased incidence of abortions.

If a suitable petfood mix is unavailable, some goat mixes and riding pony mixes will make suitable alternatives.

A simple means of giving a mixture of cereals is to give them in a bran mash, although some guinea pigs may not eat it in this form. Bran can be fed soaked in water mixed with breadcrumbs or as a soaked mix of oatmeal, wheatmeal and bran in the ratio $1:2:3$.

This can be fed daily in winter and less frequently during the summer and throughout pregnancy. In times of increased vitamin requirement (e.g. during the winter) a vitamin syrup such as Minadex can be added to the mash. As bran is low in calcium and high in phosphorus, too much during pregnancy may lead to the development of young with a poorly mineralized bone structure.

Rabbit food contains too little vitamin C and also excess vitamin D (which may lead to metastatic calcification). Some rabbit pellets for commercial rabbit production contain coccidiostats and these are unnecessary drugs for guinea pigs and have been associated with stunted growth and sporadic deaths when inadvertently fed to guinea pigs. The majority of coccidiostats are ionophores and these have a harmful effect on the natural flora of the gut, and although they may not induce diarrhoea they decrease the digestive efficiency of the guinea pig's gut and this leads to sub-optimal growth rates in the affected stock.

Aflatoxicosis

This is an infrequent condition, but it may be seen if dry food (especially maize) is stored in damp warm conditions and becomes contaminated with *Aspergillus flavus*.

Clinical signs. Varying degrees of hepatotoxicity, depending upon the amount of contaminated food consumed. Mildly affected cases will become lethargic and inappetent, whilst more acute cases will exhibit loss of coordination, convulsions and death.

Pathology. An exudative hepatitis in acute cases. Chronic cases will have cirrhotic livers.

Treatment. None.

10/ Anaesthetics and Surgical Preparations

Guinea pigs do not make particularly good anaesthetic candidates as their response to anaesthesia is extremely variable, especially if an injectable agent is used. It is always best to use a familiar anaesthetic when contemplating any form of surgery on a guinea pig; however, there are many different methods of anaesthetizing this species which have been documented in the literature and this chapter will discuss them all. Other important considerations which will contribute to the success of any procedure are careful preparation for surgery and intensive post-operative nursing.

Preparation for surgery

Before anaesthesia the guinea pig should, where possible, be fasted for at least 4 hours to minimize the likelihood of regurgitation of its stomach contents and to make its response to the anaesthetic more predictable.

If an inhalation agent is used atropine is a useful premedicant as it will reduce salivation during the anaesthetic period. A dose of 60 μg/kg should be administered by subcutaneous injection.

One of the major problems of anaesthesia in any small animal is that of heat loss during surgery, and there are several ways that this heat loss can be minimized:

1 The patient can be placed on a heat-reflective surface, e.g. 'Flectabed'.

2 The patient can be wrapped in aluminium silver foil with only the operation site exposed.

3 Extra heat can be provided by using a heat lamp above the operating table.

The patient should not be placed on a hot water bottle as this will encourage vasodilation, and therefore increase heat loss.

The operation site should be clipped and then cleaned with a suitable anti-bacterial solution, e.g. Pevidine (Tx 57) and then sprayed with surgical spirit. Do not overwet the patient as this will cause further heat loss due to the evaporation of these fluids. The cleaning solution should be used at body temperature.

The time taken for the preparation and the surgery itself should be kept to a minimum in order to cause as little stress to the patient as possible.

Depth of anaesthesia

This can be monitored by pinching either the ears or the webs of the toes. Once the responses to these stimuli disappear surgical anaesthesia has been achieved.

10.1 Inhalation anaesthetics

Induction

This is best carried out by placing a small facemask over the guinea pig's head, and supporting the guinea pig on the table by placing cupped hands over its body. During induction guinea pigs exhibit a normal squirming activity. This does not mean that they are fighting the anaesthetic and the induction concentration must not be raised as this will increase the risk of overdosage. There is a greater risk of overdosing with halothane than with methoxyflurane during induction.

Circuit

It is best to use an Ayre's T piece and a small facemask both for induction and maintenance. If a small enough facemask is unavailable one can be easily constructed from a plastic syringe case.

Halothane

This is the most commonly used anaesthetic in veterinary surgeries and it can safely be used as an anaesthetic in this species.

Induction can be achieved using a 3% concentration, with the anaesthesia maintained with a lower concentration of between 1 and 2%. This can either be used with oxygen alone or a 1 : 1 mixture of nitrous oxide and oxygen.

Methoxyflurane

If this is available it is the most suitable anaesthetic for guinea pigs.

Induction can be achieved with a 3% concentration and then adequate analgesia can be acquired by maintaining the cavy on a concentration of 0.5−1% methoxyflurane with either oxygen or nitrous oxide and oxygen as a 1 : 1 mixture.

Ether

This should not be used for guinea pigs. It is very irritant to the respiratory tract and may cause a fatal bronchospasm during induction. If ether is the only anaesthetic available the patient must be pre-medicated with atropine.

10.2   Injectable anaesthetics

All injections should be made into the quadriceps using a 23−26 gauge needle. Where possible no more than 0.3 ml should be injected at any one site, and thus in some cases the anaesthetic dose must be divided and injected equally into different muscle masses.

Hypnorm

Hypnorm (Janssen Animal Health) contains fentanyl (a morphine analgesic) and fluanisone (a neuroleptic) and it can be used to provide either sedation and light anaesthesia, or deeper anaesthesia if used in combination with diazepam (Valium, Roche).

Dose. 1 mg/kg given intramuscularly for sedation. 1 mg/kg given intramuscularly plus 2.5 mg/kg of diazepam given as an intraperitoneal injection for surgical anaesthesia. Naloxone (Narcan) given at a dose rate of 0.1 mg/kg given intraperitoneally or intramuscularly will reverse the anaesthesia.

Comment. The use of fentanyl has been associated with the development of tissue necrosis at the injection site, and also self-mutilation of the distal limb in which the injection was given.

Ketamine

Ketamine (Vetalar, Parke Davis) containing 100 mg/ml of ketamine.

Dose. 100 mg/kg given intramuscularly will provide good immobilization but little analgesia. It is a useful form of restraint for minor procedures.

Comment. The administration of ketamine has been associated with self-mutilation of the distal limb in which the injection was given.

Ketamine and Rompun

Ketamine can also be used in conjunction with Rompun (Bayer) to produce deep anaesthesia. The two drugs can be mixed together and are then best given in a divided dose intramuscularly.

Dose. Vetalar 60 mg/kg and Rompun 8 mg/kg will produce anaesthesia in 15−20 minutes. Vetalar 100 mg/kg and Rompun 4 mg/kg will produce anaesthesia in 12−15 minutes. The guinea pig should be kept in a darkened and quiet place until anaesthesia develops.

Saffan

Saffan (Coopers Pitman-Moore) contains alphaxalone and alphadolone, and the total concentration of these steroids is 12 mg/ml.

Dose. 40 mg/kg intramuscularly. This will mean a dose of 3 ml or more for an adult guinea pig and this is not often a practical dose as it is so large. Saffan is therefore not used frequently but it will produce deep sedation for minor procedures.

Pentobarbitone

The unpredictable result that intraperitoneal injection of pentobarbitone produces precludes its use in most cases. Overdose will cause respiratory depression and deep unconsciousness. It must not be used for caesarian section as it will suppress the respiratory reflexes of the fetuses.

Nembutal (Sanfoni Animal Health) contains 60 mg/ml of pentobarbitone. The dose for intraperitoneal injection is 35 mg/kg and the Nembutal is best diluted with sterile water to produce a sensibly sized injection. This will produce anaesthesia which lasts between 15 and 45 minutes. If respiratory depression is present doxapram hydrochloride (Tx 46) should be administered intramuscularly at a dose of 10–15 mg/kg.

Post-anaesthetic complications

These include respiratory infections, digestive disturbances, generalized depression and inappetance. However, many of these problems can be overcome with good nursing and post-operative care.

Immediate post-operative care

If respiration is depressed during or after surgery, doxapram hydrochloride (Tx 46) should be given at a dose of 10–15 mg/kg either subcutaneously or intramuscularly.

After surgery the patient should be kept in a warm box and allowed to recover. The optimum temperature of the recovery area should be 25–30°C (75–85°F).

15 ml of fluids (Tx 15, glucose–saline) can be administered subcutaneously. These should be gently warmed before their administration.

The convalescent patient

If the guinea pig's appetite is depressed following surgery further administration of subcutaneous fluids may be required. Alternatively fluids can be given orally via a dropper or syringe. If anorexia continues for several days after surgery the guinea pig must be given glucose in its oral fluid mixture to prevent the onset of ketosis. Oral vitamin C (20–30 mg/kg) should also be administered daily to the dehabilitated patient. Until the guinea pig begins to eat on its own it can be syringe fed with proprietary human convalescent food (e.g. Complan) or baby foods. Vetrumex (Tx 13) may also act as an effective appetite stimulant if given orally.

The patient must be constantly stimulated and encouraged. If left alone a sick guinea pig will give up quickly but intensive nursing is often quite rewarding. The presence of another guinea pig will also provide some encouragement to the convalescent guinea pig and will often stimulate it to start feeding again.

The convalescent guinea pig must be kept in warm surroundings at a constant temperature. For the individual a box in an airing cupboard will provide the perfect environment for the recovering guinea pig. Alternatively an external heat source should be provided, either in the form of a heat lamp or as a domestic light bulb. Direct contact with a hot water bottle is not recommended as there is the risk of causing burns to the guinea pig, as well as stimulating vasodilation which would be deleterious to the shocked patient. However, if the guinea pig is placed in a box with an open mesh or grid above it, a hot water-bottle can be used as an overhead heat source if placed on this 'roof' and covered with a towel.

11/ Treatments

This chapter aims to summarize all the treatments mentioned in the preceding chapters and describe their modes of administration and dosage. Each drug is coded with a treatment (Tx) number for easy cross reference.

All the doses are given in milligrams (mg) or millilitres (ml) per kg. As a rough guide-line an adult guinea pig weighs 1 kg, although some of the larger types may weigh up to 1400 g. The birth weight is between 75 and 100 g and their weight gain is approximately 4 g/day until they reach their adult weight at 8 months of age.

Routes of drug administration

Subcutaneous injection. This can be given under the skin at the scruff of the neck or, for larger volumes of injection, under the skin overlying the thorax. Up to 10 ml can be administered in this way. A 23–26 gauge needle should be used.

Intramuscular injection. This can be administered into the quadriceps muscles using a 23–26 gauge needle. The maximum volume given at one site is 0.3 ml. If a series of daily injections is to be given alternate hindlegs should be used on subsequent days.

Intraperitoneal injection. The guinea pig is best held supported under its forelegs and bottom and positioned on its back with its head held slightly lower than its hindquarters to allow the stomach and intestines to fall forward. The needle should be inserted to the right of the midline 2.5 cm in front of the pubis, and directed forwards at an angle of 45°. Up to 15 ml can be administered using a 23–25 gauge needle.

Intravenous injection. The veins of a guinea pig are very small and dosing via this route is difficult. The largest and most accessible veins are the ear veins and the bracheocephalic vein.

Oral dosing. This is the most frequently used route for drug administration used in general practice as it is usually the most practicable. However it is frequently associated with antibiotic toxicity as antibiotics given orally have a direct and undesirable effect on the natural gut flora (see later). It is very important to use oral antibiosis with great caution and only when it is really necessary.

Drops of liquid can be placed on the tongue via a dropper or a syringe. One drop from a 2 ml syringe is equivalent to 0.02 ml.

It is not generally recommended to mix antibiotics in the drinking water as the water intake of a sick guinea pig may be markedly reduced, whilst healthy individuals in the same pen may take in large and often toxic amounts of the antibiotic. An exception to this is if a colony problem is being treated (e.g. *Coccidium*).

Stomach tube. A pliable rubber or plastic tube with a diameter of 1.5−6 mm is recommended. The disadvantage of this method is that the guinea pig may need to be anaesthetized for this procedure and this is undesirable for most weak or debilitated patients.

Antibiotics

Antibiotics must be administered with caution as the guinea pig is very sensitive to the toxic effects of many of the commonly used antibiotics. This toxicity occurs because the antibiotics destroy the natural gut bacteria which enables the overgrowth of *Clostridia* spp., especially *Clostridium difficile*, as well as other Gram-negative species. This overgrowth causes a fatal enterotoxaemia leading to diarrhoea and death between 3 and 7 days after the administration of the antibiotic.

Antibiotics with a narrow spectrum of activity appear to be the most toxic, especially if the activity is against Gram-positive organisms. Antibiotics that have known toxic activity are:
- Ampicillin.
- Bacitracin.
- Erythromycin.
- Lincocin.
- Penicillin.
- Streptomycin.
- Tylosin.
- Tetracycline.

The risk of inducing enterotoxaemia is highest when using oral preparations as they have a direct effect on the bacterial flora of the gut. The incidence of side-effects are lower with parenterally administered antibiotics. Care must also be taken if using topical preparations as they can produce the same syndrome if licked at by the affected guinea pig or its inmates.

The risk of toxicity can be reduced if the antibiotic is given concurrently with a probiotic (see later).

The simultaneous administration of a vitamin B complex may also help prevent these undesirable side-effects.

Before treating any individual with antibiotics one must be certain that the benefits outweigh the potentially harmful consequences.

11.1   Antibiotics

Tx 1. Cephaloridine

Ceporin (Coopers Pitman-Moore)

This antibiotic against *Streptococcus zooepidemicus* at a dose of 25 mg/kg intramuscularly is often recommended in the literature. However this antibiotic has been superseded by another broad-spectrum cephalosporin, cephalexin (Ceporex, Coopers Pitman-Moore).

Tx 2. Cephalexin

Ceporex (Coopers Pitman-Moore)

This contains 180 mg/ml cephalexin.

Dose. 50 mg/kg by intramuscular injection daily. This approximates to a dose of 0.25 ml/kg.

This is now used in place of Cephaloridine (see above). The recommended dose should be given for 14 days when treating *Streptococcus zooepidemicus*.

Tx 3. Chloramphenicol

Chloramphenicol injectable suspension (Willows Francis)

This contains 150 mg/ml of chloramphenicol.

Dose. 20 mg/kg injected intramuscularly daily. This approximates to a dose of 0.15 ml/kg.

Chloramphenicol is the drug of choice for treating cases with central nervous system involvement as it readily crosses the blood—brain barrier.

Tx 4. Metronidazole

Torgyl (Rhône Mérieux)

This contains 5 mg/ml metronidazole.

Dose. 20 mg/kg once daily. This is equivalent to 4 ml/kg. It can be given orally, mixed with food or water, or injected subcutaneously. The major disadvantage of this is the large quantity of drug that must be injected but the dose can be split and administered at two different sites, which will also lead to a faster rate of its absorption.

Tx 5. Neomycin

Neobiotic Aquadrops (Upjohn Ltd)

These contain 50 mg/ml of neomycin and 0.25 mg/ml of meth-scopolamine bromide. The latter is an anti-cholinesterase and helps combat bacterial enteritis.

Dose. The dose per guinea pig is 5 mg/kg twice daily. The drops are diluted 1:4 with water (1 part aquadrops:4 parts water) to produce a solution containing 10 mg/ml of neomycin and the dose is 0.5 ml/kg twice daily. This should be given orally.

Neomycin is poorly absorbed from the digestive tract and if it is used to treat infections elsewhere in the body it may fail to reach therapeutic levels at its required site of action. It is however, a very useful antibiotic for the treatment of diarrhoea and is a component of Neosulphentrin suspension (see later).

Tx 6. Nitrofuratoin

This is a human drug which can be used in cases of cystitis. Furadantin 50 mg (Norwich Eaton) contains 50 mg of nitrofuratoin.

Dose. One tablet (50 mg/kg) a day for 3 days.

Tx 7. Sulphadimidine

Sulphamezathine solution 33% (Coopers Pitman-Moore)

This contains 0.33 g/ml sulphadimidine sodium.

Dose. The solution can be diluted 1:1 with water and 3 ml/kg given three times daily by oral administration. This is equivalent to a dose of 0.5 g/kg of sulphadimidine sodium three times daily.

The treatment should not be continued for longer than 5 days.

Alternatively the drinking water can be replaced by a 0.2% solution of sulphadimidine sodium (1 ml of sulphamezathine 33%:150 ml water).

This sulphonamide can be given against the majority of infections and is particularly useful in the treatment of coccidiosis.

Tx 8. Tetracyclines

Although this class of drug has reported toxicity, it has widespread use in general practice with few side-effects. It is, however, recommended that this drug is used with great caution, and preferably in conjunction with a probiotic.

Tetracyclines should only be given orally by dropper and never mixed with the drinking water as there is the risk that in-contact healthy individuals may consume large and toxic amounts of antibiotics as they fulfil their daily water intake.

Dose. 50 mg/kg/day in three divided doses. Alternatively 5 mg/kg can be injected intramuscularly twice a day.

Tx 9. Trimethoprim

Tribrissen injection 24% (Coopers Pitman-Moore)

This contains 40 mg/ml trimethoprim and 200 mg/ml sulphadiazine sodium.

Dose. 0.5 ml/kg injected subcutaneously daily.

Tribrissen 20 tablets (Coopers Pitman-Moore)

These contain 20 mg trimethoprim and 100 mg sulphadiazine sodium.

Dose. These can be crushed to a powder and a quarter of a tablet given daily to an adult guinea pig. Alternatively the dose can be divided and an eighth of a tablet given twice daily.

Borgal 7.5% (Hoechst)

This contains 12.5 mg/ml trimethoprim and 62.5 mg/ml sulphadoxine.

Dose. 0.5 ml/kg daily by subcutaneous or intramuscular injection.

11.2   Probiotics

These can be given at the same time as the antibiotic to help protect the gut from the damaging effects which occur as the intestinal bacterial flora are destroyed. Probiotics provide a supply of these natural flora.

Tx 10. Enterodex

Enterodex (Vydex, Animal Health Ltd)

Give 1 gm (¼ teaspoon) mixed with food or a little water once a day.

Tx 11. Live natural yogurt

This contains *Acidophilus* and *Lactobacillus*. A few drops can be given from a teaspoon twice daily.

Tx 12. Probios

Probios ruminant granules (Deosan Ltd)

This is a dried fermentation product of selected strains of beneficial bacteria together with yeast culture, vegetable oil and preservatives. It is formulated for ruminants to provide naturally occurring bacteria and added vitamins to the digestive tract.

Dose. A quarter of a teaspoon mixed with a little water daily.

Tx 13. Vetrumex

This is a cattle preparation which contains bacteria necessary for repopulating the rumen. It also acts as an appetite stimulant in cavies as well as cattle and can be given for this purpose even when antibiotics are not being used.

Dose. A quarter or half a teaspoon mixed with a little water or rosehip syrup daily. It can be administered twice daily if necessary.

11.3   Fluid therapy

Tx 14. Normal saline 0.9%

In cases of dehydration this fluid can be administered subcutaneously. 10 ml can be given at any one site in the skin overlying the thorax. Up to 20 ml can be given on any one occasion.

Tx 15. Glucose−saline

5% glucose with 0.9% saline. This is particularly useful in cases of ketosis or anorexia. It can be used post-operatively to provide rehydration and energy. It can be administered subcutaneously and up to 10 ml can be given at any one site.

Tx 16. Lectade

Lectade (SmithKline Beecham)

This preparation is used for oral rehydration. As it contains dextrose it is also very useful as a preventative measure for pregnancy toxaemia if it is used to replace the drinking water.

Lectade is available in powder or liquid form. The latter is the more convenient to use and should be used at the dilution of 20 ml liquid Lectade to 250 ml water.

11.4   Anti-fungal agents

Tx 17. Benzuldazic acid

Defungit (Hoechst) is the sodium salt of this acid and it can be applied externally as a 0.5% solution every 3 days.

Tx 18. Griseofulvin

Grisovin powder and Grisovin tablets (Coopers Pitman-Moore)

The powder contains 7.5% griseofulvin, and the tablets 125 mg griseofulvin.

Dose. 25 mg/kg daily. This can be achieved by administering a fifth of a tablet daily, or by incorporating the powder in the feed at a rate of 10 g/kg of dry feed (equivalent to 0.75 mg/kg griseofulvin). This assumes that the average daily intake of dry food is 30 g/kg bodyweight.

If Grisovin is used to treat an individual guinea pig it is best given orally, and in these circumstances an eighth of a teaspoon of Grisovin can be mixed with a small amount of an unsaturated fatty acid supplement (e.g. 0.5 ml Norderm, Norden Laboratories) and given daily.

Comment. Griseofulvin should not be administered to the pregnant animal as it is teratogenic.

Tx 19. Tolnaftate 1%

Tinaderm-M cream

This is a human anti-fungal preparation which can be applied to fungal lesions twice a day until they resolve.

Other topical preparations, e.g. Panalog cream, contain the anti-fungal nystatin as one of their components.

11.5 Anti-diarrhoeal preparations

Tx 20. Kaolin

This substance is available in several preparations, either on its own or in combination with other therapeutic agents.

Tx 21. Kaopectate V (Upjohn Ltd)

This preparation contains kaolin alone.

Dose. 0.2 ml given 3−4 times daily.

Tx 22. KLN

This is an infant anti-diarrhoeal preparation, containing light kaolin, fruit pectin, oil of peppermint and sodium citrate.

Dose. 3−4 drops three times daily.

Tx 23. Kaolin−morphine

This combination is useful for painful colics.

Dose. 0.2 ml given three times daily.

Tx 24. Neosulphentrin suspension (Willows Francis)

This also contains a combination of neomycin and sulphonamides.

Dose. 0.3 ml three times daily. This is useful if an infectious enteritis is suspected, but it must be given with a probiotic to replace the natural gut flora which will be upset by the Neo-sulphentrin.

11.6   Topical preparations

Tx 25. Dermisol

Dermisol (SmithKline Beecham)

This cream contains propylene glycol, malic acid, benzoic acid and salicylic acid. It promotes healing by removing dead and necrotic tissue from affected areas and also has anti-bacterial properties.

Dose. Dermisol can be applied to affected areas 2−3 times daily until the condition resolves.

The same constituents also make up a multi-cleanse solution which is useful to remove necrotic tissue and promote healing.

Tx 26. Kamillosan

This is a herbal preparation which is particularly useful in the treatment of sore nipples. It has the added advantage of being safe to use even when the young are suckling. A little can be applied to the affected nipples 2−3 times daily.

Tx 27. Panolog cream

Panolog cream (Ciba-Geigy)

This contains triamcinolone acetonide (potent steroid), neomycin and thiostrepton (antibiotics), and nystatin (anti-fungal).

It is a useful preparation for dermatitis and mixed infections which are accompanied by severe inflammation and pruritus. It can be applied up to three times a day. It is particularly useful for treating scabs around the mouth.

Tx 28. Vetsovate

Vetsovate (Coopers Pitman-Moore)

This contains 0.1% betamethasone (steroid) and 0.5% neomycin (antibiotic). It is useful for bacterial infections accompanied by inflammation and pruritus. It can be applied to the affected area 2−3 times a day.

11.7   Eye preparations

Antibiotic only

These should be used when there is corneal damage. There are various preparations available.

Tx 29. Chloramphenicol

Chloromycetin ophthalmic ointment 1% (Parke Davis). Apply 4−6 times a day.

Tx 30. Cephalonium

Cepravin eye ointment (Coopers Pitman-Moore). Apply 1−2 times a day.

Antibiotic and steroid

These can be used for conjunctivitis where there is no accompanying corneal damage.

Tx 31. Chloramphenicol

Chloromycetin hydrocortisone ophthalmic ointment (Parke Davis). Apply 4–6 times a day.

Tx 32. Neobiotic HC

Neomycin and hydrocortisone (Upjohn Ltd). This preparation is formulated as readily flowing drops and is therefore easier to administer than creams to some patients. Apply 3–6 times daily.

Tx 33. Panolog ophthalmic (Ciba-Geigy)

This has the same components as the cream (see Tx 26) and therefore has anti-fungal activity too. Although it contains steroid it is very effective in the acute stages of corneal ulceration if this is accompanied by marked conjunctival inflammation.

Apply 2–3 times daily initially, then less frequently as the condition improves.

Panalog has been applied to eyes without any obvious side effects if the ophthalmic ointment is unavailable.

Steroid only

Tx 34. Betsolan eye and ear drops (Coopers Pitman-Moore)

Apply 1 drop 4–6 times daily as required.

11.8 Ectoparasitic preparations

Tx 35. Seleen

Seleen (Sanfoni Animal Health Ltd)

This is a yellow suspension containing 1% selenium sulphide. It has both anti-parasitic and anti-fungal properties, and is useful for the simultaneous treatment of dermatomycoses and external parasites.

It is also beneficial if extensive seborrhea is present.

The whole guinea pig should be wetted, and the shampoo applied and worked to a lather. The shampoo should be left on the coat for at least 5 minutes before rinsing. Treatment can be repeated weekly as necessary, or more frequently if the condition is severe.

Tx 36. Ivermectin

Ivermectin injection for cattle (Merck, Sharpe & Dohme Ltd). This product is not licensed for guinea pigs and must be used with care. It is however a very effective ectoparasitic agent.

The dose is 200 μg/kg and this can be repeated at 10–14 day intervals as necessary. The dose of the cattle injection is 0.02 ml/kg, so it is best diluted 1 : 10 with water for injection to produce a more convenient dose of 0.2 ml which should be administered subcutaneously.

Alternatively the drug can be given orally in its undiluted form. One drop from a 2 ml syringe is equivalent to 200 μg and up to 2 drops can be administered to an adult cavy with no adverse side-effects.

Trials at the Cambridge Cavy Trust have shown that larger doses of ivermectin (cattle injection) can be given without any adverse side-effects. Their recommendations are as follows:
- Age 3 weeks to 3 months: 0.1 ml by subcutaneous injection. Oral dosing not recommended.
- Age 3 months onward: 0.2 ml by subcutaneous injection. One drop given orally.

Ivermectin has been administered safely to pregnant sows.

Tx 37. Tetmosol

Tetmosol (ICI Pharmaceuticals)

This is a human scabies preparation which contains monosulfiram as its active ingredient.

It should be diluted 1 : 72 with water. This approximates to one tablespoon of Tetmosol to a litre of water. The whole guinea pig should be dipped in this solution which should be worked into the coat. The guinea pig should not be rinsed but allowed to dry. The solution may stain the coat of light-coloured individuals a yellow colour for a few days subsequent to treatment which can be repeated fortnightly.

Tetmosol is especially effective for the treatment of mange but will effectively remove other ectoparasites too.

Tx 38. Quellada

Quellada veterinary shampoo (Stafford-Miller Ltd)

The active ingredient is gamma benzene hexachloride, and it is a very effective ectoparasitic preparation. The guinea pig must be wetted with water and then Quellada is applied as a shampoo, worked well into a lather and then rinsed off after 3–4 minutes and the guinea pig is then dried well. This treatment can be repeated weekly.

11.9 Endoparasitic preparations

Tx 39. Metronidazole

Flagyl suspension (May and Baker Pharmaceuticals)

This contains 40 mg/ml of active metronidazole. This is used to treat diseases caused by anaerobic organisms and is also effective against *Trichomonas* spp.

The dose is 20 mg/kg daily given in the drinking water for 7–10 days. The correct dose will be given if 1 ml of Flagyl suspension is mixed with 150 ml of drinking water.

The active ingredient of Torgyl (Tx 4) is also metronidazole.

Tx 40. Piperazine

Antepar elixir (Wellcome Medical Division)

This will effectively control nematodes at a dose of piperazine 3 mg/ml of water. Antepar contains 150 mg piperazine per millilitre and should be diluted 1 ml of Antepar to 50 ml of water, and this solution used to replace the drinking water for a day.

Tx 41. Praziquantel

Droncit (Bayer)

This will effectively control cestodes at a dose of 5–10 mg/kg orally or 5 mg/kg given by subcutaneous injection.

Tx 42. Sulphadimidine

Sulphamezathine 33% (Coopers Pitman-Moore)

This is a useful preparation for the treatment of coccidiosis. It is given in the drinking water at concentration of 2% for 5 days. This concentration will be achieved by diluting 10 ml of sulphamethazine 33% with 165 ml water.

11.10   Miscellaneous treatments

Tx 43. Atropine

Atropine sulphate injection (Animalcare Ltd) contains 600 µg/ml.

Dose for premedication: 60 µg/kg; and for organophosphate poisoning: 100 µg/kg. Both these should be given by subcutaneous injection.

Tx 44. Betamethasone

Betsolan (Coopers Pitman-Moore)

This is a steroid preparation with powerful anti-inflammatory properties. It can be used in the treatment of pregnancy toxaemia, and the glucogenic effect it produces will last for several days.

Dose. 0.1–0.2 ml given by subcutaneous or intramuscular injection.

Comment. Steroids should not be administered in early pregnancy as they have been shown to cause fetal abnormalities. There is also a risk that they may cause abortion in late pregnancy, but their beneficial effect in the treatment of ketosis outweighs this slight risk.

Tx 45. Dexamethasone

Dexafort (Intervet UK Ltd)

This combination of long- and short-acting steroid produces a rapid and long-lasting glucogenic effect and is very important in the treatment of pregnancy toxaemia (ketosis). This drug also has a long-lasting anti-inflammatory and anti-pruritic effect and can be useful in the treatment of skin conditions which are accompanied by intense pruritus.

Dose. In cases of ketosis 0.1 ml should be administered intramuscularly. For the treatment of any other conditions the same dose can be administered subcutaneously.

Comment. The same comments apply for dexamethasone as for betamethasone (see above).

Tx 46. Doxapram hydrochloride

Dopram-V (Willows Francis)

This contains 20 mg/ml of doxapram hydrochloride, and it is a useful respiratory stimulant.

Dose. 10−15 mg/kg by subcutaneous or intramuscular injection.

Tx 47. Hexetidine

Hexocil (Parke Davis) contains 0.5% hexetidine as a shampoo.

It has anti-bacterial and anti-fungal properties, and is especially useful in cases with severe seborrhoea of fungal origin. When used to treat fungal conditions it should be in contact with the skin for up to 2 hours before rinsing.

Tx 48. Oxytocin

Oxytocin-S (Intervet UK Ltd)

One ml contains 10 oxytocin units. The dose to stimulate uterine contractions and milk let-down is 1−2 units, i.e. 0.1−0.2 ml injected intramuscularly.

Tx 49. Primidone

Mysoline suspension (Coopers Pitman-Moore) contains 50 mg/ml primidone.

Dose. 0.5 ml/kg twice daily orally.

Tx 50. Tarlite

Tarlite is a tar-based shampoo which is of particular use in cases of seborrhoea, whatever the primary cause of the condition.

It should be used as a shampoo, and applied to the coat once it is wet and then left on the coat for 2−3 minutes before it is rinsed off well. Treatments can be repeated weekly for as often as is necessary.

Tx 51. Diazepam

Valium (Roche)

A dose of 1−2 mg/kg can be given intramuscularly to produce a calming effect in cases with intense pruritus or to those mothers which are initially very apprehensive of their young.

11.11   Vitamin preparations

Tx 52. Abidec drops

Abidec drops (Parke Davis)

These drops contain vitamins A, C, D and vitamin B complex. Up to 2 drops (0.1 ml) can be given daily to an adult, the dose for a young animal is 1 drop per day.

Abidec drops are useful to ensure adequate vitamins for convalescent animals. Two drops contain 10 mg of vitamin C which is adequate for maintenance of a guinea pig weighing 1 kg. If further vitamin C is required it must be included as an extra supplement.

Tx 53. Collo-Cal D

Collo-Cal D (C-Vet) contains 0.75% w/v colloidal calcium oleate and 70 iu/ml of vitamin D.

Dose. 0.5 ml/kg orally once a day.

Tx 54. Redoxon

Soluble vitamin C tablets containing 1000 mg. One tablet should be dissolved in 8 litres of water to produce the required concentration. Tablets are therefore best divided and added to smaller amounts of water. In instances of increased requirements (e.g. pregnancy) one 1000 mg tablet can be dissolved in 5 litres of water.

If vitamin C is being given to treat a clinical case of deficiency it should be given at a rate of 100 mg/kg. In this instance a tenth of a tablet can be dissolved in a very small amount of water and administered orally.

The diluted solution should be given in glass dishes or drinking bottles with stainless steel nozzles. The breakdown of ascorbic acid is accelerated if it comes into contact with any other metals. Alternatively the required amount (80 ml of the diluted solution) can be mixed in a bran mash.

Tx 55. Vitamin B$_{12}$

This is a very useful vitamin for use in convalescense, and in cases of debilitation of inappetance.

Dose. 0.25 ml of vitamin B$_{12}$ 250 µg given by subcutaneous or intramuscular injection. Treatment can be repeated weekly if necessary.

11.12   Cleansing solutions

Tx 56. Hydrogen peroxide

This is very useful for flushing out wounds and abscesses. It should be used at a concentration of 3%.

Tx 57. Povidone-iodine

Povidine antiseptic solution (BK Veterinary Products)

This contains 1% active iodine and it has anti-microbial action against bacteria, fungi, yeasts and some viruses.

It can be used in its concentrated form on wounds, mange, fungal and bacterial infections. It can also be used dilute as a bathing solution, mixed 1 : 5 with water.

Tx 58. Savlon

Savlon Veterinary Concentrate (Coopers Pitman-Moore)

This has antiseptic and anti-bacterial properties and it is a useful skin cleaning agent. It should be diluted 1 : 30 in water for use.

Tx 59. Salt solution

The most readily available all purpose bathing solution is a teaspoon of common salt dissolved in a pint of warm water.

12/ Zoonotic Aspects

Guinea pigs are generally kept in close association with humans, as the majority of them are children's pets or kept by the hobbyist for breeding and exhibiting. Although there are several potential zoonotic organisms which may affect guinea pigs they are seldom associated with human disease.

Ringworm

This is the most common zoonosis as the fungal spores are transferred when the guinea pig is handled. The most frequently isolated dermatophyte is *Trichophyton mentagrophytes*, and lesions on the owner are usually found on the hands and arms.

Proven or suspect cases of ringworm should only be handled for the administration of treatment, and gloves should be worn for this procedure. Any spores on in-contact bedding can be destroyed by burning, and the hutch can be cleaned with a 2% formalin solution, or with a hexetidine preparation (Tx 47).

Mange

Mange caused by *Trixacarus caviae* is probably the most frequent skin complaint of guinea pigs. However, human skin disease caused by this mite is very rare, presumably because this mite is a burrowing mite and not immediately accessible for transmission. Extra precautions are not usually necessary during the treatment of affected individuals.

Salmonella

This organism has the most public health significance, but thankfully it is a rare pathogen for guinea pigs. However, when *Salmonella* spp. are isolated the whole caviary should be depopulated. Healthy animals which are not in-contact can be removed and isolated, but affected animals and those which recover should be destroyed.

Recovered animals are likely to become carriers and therefore per-petuate the disease.

All premises, feeding and drinking utensils should be thoroughly disinfected with a 5% formalin solution or other approved disinfectant and all bedding and hay destroyed by burning.

Yersinia (pseudotuberculosis)

This disease is also rarely seen in guinea pigs. However, when diagnosed all affected animals should be destroyed and all premises and utensils well disinfected.

Allergic responses to guinea pigs

Some owners may develop asthma-like symptoms after being in close association with guinea pigs. The allergen may be their hair or skin debris, but more commonly is the hay and the owner develops a condition akin to 'farmer's lung'. Avoiding the use of mouldy or dusty hay, and the wearing of a facemask whilst in the caviary should minimize the symptoms.

Other allergy symptoms which have been reported in laboratory technicians and other personnel working in close association with guinea pigs, are rhinitis and skin rashes.

Appendix: Miscellaneous Physiological Data

Body temperature (rectal thermometer)	38.3−40°C (100−104°F)
Heart rate	230−320/minute
Respiration rate	90−150/minute
Tidal volume	2−5 ml/kg
Blood volume	6% of body weight
Life expectancy	up to 8 years, usually 4−5 years
Environmental temperature	20−22°C (optimum performance)
	15−18°C (acceptable average)

Digestive parameters

Food intake	6 g per 100 g body weight of which 2−4 g is dry food. They eat 8% of their body weight as dried food
Water intake	85 ml/day (average adult). Approximately 8 ml/100 g body weight
First eat solid food	2−4 days old

Reproductive parameters

Sexual maturity (female)	4−6 weeks
Sexual maturity (male)	4−6 weeks
Female breeding age	4−5 months, weight 500 g
Male breeding age	3−5 months, weight 550 g
Oestrus cycle	15−17 days
Ovulation	Spontaneous — approximately 10 hours after onset of oestrus
Gestation period	59−72 days (depending upon litter size)
Litter size	1−6 (average 3)
Birthweight	75−100 g
Breeding life of female	4−5 years
Breeding life of male	5 years or longer
Lactation period	3 weeks
Weaning age	3 weeks

Haematology

Blood sampling. Small samples can be collected by overclipping a toe-nail 0.25 ml can be obtained by venesection of the marginal ear vein.

Blood volume (ml/kg body weight)	75
Haematocrit	37−48
Haemaglobin (g/dl blood)	11−17.2
RBC count (per ml)	4.5−7000 000
WBC count (per ml)	3.2−15 000 000
Neutrophils	28−44% (average 37%)
Lymphocytes	39−72% (average 56%)
Eosinophils	1−5%
Monocytes	3−12%
Basophils	0−3%

Further Reading

Anderson, L. (1987) Guinea pig husbandry and medicine. *Veterinary Clinics of North America* 1045–1059.

Axelrod, J. (1980) *Breeding Guinea pigs.* TFH Publications, USA.

Buckland, M.D., Hall, L. *et al.* (1981) *A Guide to Laboratory Animal Technology.* Heinemann, USA.

Cooper, G. and Schiller, R.L. (1975) *Anatomy of the Guinea Pig.* Harvard Press.

Elward, M. (1980) *Encyclopedia of Guinea Pigs.* TFH Publications, USA.

Flecknell, P. (1983) Restraint, anaesthesia and treatment of children's pets. *In Practice* May, 85–95.

Flecknell, P. (1985) *Guinea Pigs. Manual of Exotic Pets.* BSAVA 36–44.

Harkness, J.E. and Wagner, J.E. (1989) *The Biology and Medicine of Rabbits and Rodents.* Lea and Febiger, Philadelphia.

Hime, J.M. and O'Donoghue, P.N. (1979) *Handbook of Diseases of Laboratory Animals.* Heinemann.

Hutchinson, P. (1978) *Guinea Pigs, Their Care and Breeding.* K and R Books Ltd.

Lawrence, K. (1987) Facts and data to help the treatment of smaller domestic pets. *The Henston Veterinary Vade Mecum.* 337–340.

The Merck Veterinary Manual (1979) Merck and Co. Inc., New Jersey, USA.

Sebesteny, A. (1976) Diseases of guinea pigs. *Veterinary Record* **98**, 418–423.

Turner, I. (1981) *Exhibition and Pet Cavies.* Spur Publications.

University Federation of Animal Welfare (1976) *The UFAW Handbook of Care and Management of Laboratory Animals.* Churchill Livingstone.

Wagner, J.E. and Manning, P.J. (1976) *Biology of the Guinea Pig.* Academic Press, New York.

Williams, C.S.F. (1979) Guinea pigs and rabbits. *Veterinary Clinics of North America* 9(3), 487–497.

Index

Abidec drops 118
  diarrhoea and 59
  orphans and 33
  pneumonia and 47
  post-natal sores and 7
abortion 23–4
  enteritis and 47
  pneumonia and 47
  protein and 96
  steroids and 116
  temperature and 85
abscesses 11–12, 119
  in the neck 78
  in pregnancy 47
  tooth root 76
Absidia corymbifera 57
Absidia ramosa 57
Acidophilus 108
aflatoxicosis 96
agalactica 31–2
aggression 81, 82
allergic responses
  of guinea pigs 69
  to guinea pigs 122
alopecia 8–10
  during pregnancy 32
amniotic fluid, premature loss of 27
amphotericin B 2
ampicillin 104
anaesthetics 97–102
  complications after 101
  depth of 98
  inhalation 98–100
    circuit 98
    induction 98
  injectable 99–100
anal fold dermatitis 13
anorexia 60
Antepar elixir 115
antibiotic/steroid eye ointment 113
antibiotics 105–8
  administration 104–5
  toxicity 104–5
anti-diarrhoeal preparations 110–11

anti-fungal agents 109–10
aphlatoxicosis 57
apple 91
ascaridae 56
Aspergillus flavus 57, 96
asthma 47
astringents 93
atrophy *see* wasting disease
atropine 97, 116
aural haematoma 72

basal cell tumour 13
beetroot 90
beetroot ruttle 48
Bemax, post natal sores and 7
bent leg 62
benzoic acid 111
benzuldazic acid 2, 109–10
betamethasone 112, 116, 117
  cerebellar disease and 83
  heatstroke and 86
  pregnancy toxaemia and 22
Betsolan eye and ear drops 69, 72,
    113, 116
blowfly myiasis 14
boils 12–13
Bordetella spp. 37, 47, 66
Bordetella bronchiseptica 24, 47, 48
Borgal 108
bramble leaves 93
breeding 18
broccoli 90
broken back 6–7, 94
brussel sprouts 90
bull backed fetus 27

cabbage 90
caesarean section 28–9, 100
calamine lotion 8
calcium supplementation
  during pregnancy 22
  dystocia and 27
  eclampsia and 32
Candida albicans 50, 69

carrot 91
castor oil cream
  polyuria and 41
  urine-scalding and 11
castration 38
cataracts 44, 71
  congenital 70
cauliflower 91
celery 91
cephalexin 78, 105
cephalosporin 47, 105
Cepravin eye ointment 68, 69, 112
cerebellar disease 82−3
cerebral vascular accident 83
cervical lymphadenitis 11, 78−9
Cestoda 54−5, 116
chewing 10, 87
Chirodiscoides caviae 5, 6
chlamydial neonatal conjunctivitis 70
chloramphenicol 52, 105−6, 112, 113
chloromycetin eye ointment 113
Chloromycetin hydrocortisone 68,
  114
cleansing solutions 119−20
cleavers 93
cleft palate 76−7
Clostridium spp. 53, 58, 104
Clostridium difficile 104
coccidiosis 55−6, 107, 116
Coccidium spp. 50, 54, 55, 104
cod-liver oil
  'broken back' and 6
  osteoporosis and 64
  skin lesions after parturition and 8
  vitamin D overdose and 75, 87
colic 59
Collo-Cal D 64, 118
coltsfoot 93
Complan 101
congenital cataracts 70
conjunctivitis 68, 69, 113
  chlamydial neonatal 70
convulsions 2
coprophagia 50−1
corneal ulceration 68, 69, 113
corns 62
Corynebacterium pyogenes 11, 30
coughing 46
cryptosporidium 55
crystalluria 42
cyst, epidermoid (sebaceous) 11
cystic ovaries 37

cystitis
  haematuria and 41
  infertility and 36, 41
  nitrofurantoin 106
  penile urethra occlusion and 42
cytomegalovirus 78

dandelions 93
deficiency disease 88−90
demodex 5
dermatitis
  anal fold 13
  preputial 35
  solar 73
Dermisol 111
  abscesses and 12
  anal fold dermatitis and 13
  broken back and 6
  corns, pressure points and 62
  mastitis and 30
  overgrown toe-nails and 61
  polyuria and 41
  preputial prolapse and 35
Dexafort 117
dexamethasone 22, 117
diabetes mellitus
  polydipsia and 40
  wasting disease and 76, 89
diarrhoea
  antibiotic-induced 58−9
  infectious causes 51−4
  non-infectious causes of 56−8
  parasitic causes 54−6
Diazepam 99, 118
  fits and 82
  mange and 4
  rejection of the young and 30
dichlorvos, fur mite and 6
digestive system 49−60
  anatomy 49−50
  physiology 50
docks 93
doxapram hydrochloride 100−1, 117
Droncit 116
drug administration, routes of 103−5
  intramuscular injection 103
  intraperitoneal injection 103
  intravenous injection 103
  oral dosing 104
  stomach tube 104
  subcutaneous injection 103
dystocia 26−7, 94

ear 72−4
Echinoccus granulosus 55
eclampsia 32
ectoparasitic preparations 113−15
Eimeria caviae 55, 56
endoparasitic preparations 115−16
Entamoeba spp. 54
Enterobacteriaceae 11, 30
Enterodex 102
enterotoxaemia 58, 82, 98, 99
entropion 70
epidermoid cyst 11
epilepsy 81−2
epistaxis 45
erythromycin 98
Escherichia coli 42, 50, 54
ether 99
Eucalyptus oil, pneumonia and 47
evening primrose oil 6, 64
eye 68−72
    injuries 85
    preparations 112−13

Farex 33
fatty eye 71
feet 61
Fenbendazole, ascaridae and 56
fentanyl 99
fits 3, 82
Flagyl suspension 115
Flectabed 97
Fluanisone 99
fluid therapy 109
fly strike 14
food
    values of cultivated crops 90−1
    values of fruit 91
    see also nutrition
foreign bodies
    in the eye 68
    in the neck 79
fostering 34
fractures 66
frusemide, pneumonia and 47
fur mite 5, 6
Furadantin 106
Fusiformis 79

gamma benzene hexachloride 4, 115
gastric torsion 59
Gliricola porcelli 6
glucose-saline 22, 29, 57, 101, 109

goosegrass 93
grass 93
grease gland 12−13
griseofulvin 1−2, 110
groundsel 93, 94
Gyropus ovalis 6

haematoma, aural 72
haematuria 41
haemorrhage
    intra-uterine 24
    post-partum 28
hair chewing 10, 87
halothane 98
heatstroke 85, 86
hexetidine 2, 117, 121
Hexocil 117
housing 84−6
    environment 85
    flooring 84−5
    hygiene 85
    shared with rabbits 10
    size of accommodation 84
hydrogen peroxide 12, 79, 119
hydronephrosis 43
Hymenoplesis spp. 55
hyperphosphataemia 65
hypervitaminosis C 77, 87
hypervitaminosis D 8, 64, 75, 87
Hypnorm 99
hypocalcaemia 65
    dystocia and 27
    in pregnancy 22

impaction of the rectum 51
infant mortality, griseofulvin and 2
infertility 34−8
    boar 34−5
    cystitis and 36, 41
    sow 35−6
    treatment 36−8
intussusception 59
intra-uterine haemorrhage 24
ivermectin 114
    demodex and 5
    mange and 3, 4

Kamillosan 31, 112
kaolin 59, 110
kaolin−morphine 59, 111
Kaopectate V 110−11
ketamine 99−100

ketoacidosis 22
Ketol, pregnancy toxaemia and 21
ketosis 116, 117
    eclampsia and 32
    fits and 82
    obesity and 22
Klebsiella pneumoniae 47
KLN 58, 111
Konakion 28, 90

Lactobacillus spp. 50, 108
Lasix solution 47
laxatives 93
Lectade 109
    diarrhoea and 57
    pregnancy toxaemia and 22
lens luxation 71
lettuce 91
lice 5−6
lighting, reproduction and 37
Lincocin 63, 104
lincomycin 63
lips 77−8
liver disease
    alopecia and 9
    fits and 82
    seborrhoea and 8

malic acid 111
malnutrition, mange and 5
malocclusions 76
mange 2, 3−5, 8, 115, 120, 121
mange mite 22, 82
mastitis 30
metastatic calcification 64−5, 89, 96
methoxyflurane 98−99
methscopolamine bromide 106
metritis 37
metronidazole 54, 106, 115
microphthalmia 27, 68
microphthalmic whites 68
Microsporum gypseum 1
middle ear disease 73−4
milk, composition of 33−4
milk thistle 93
milky ocular discharge 71
Minadex 96
mineral deficiency 7
mirror eye 70
miscarriage 23−4
monosulfiram 114
mouth 74−8

multivitamins
    alopecia and 8
    diarrhoea and 60
muscular dystrophy 65, 88
musculoskeletal system 61−7
mutilation
    of the young 28
    self- 4, 7, 99, 100
mycoses 2
Mysoline 4, 118

Naloxone 111
Narcan 111
nasal discharge 45
neck 78−80
nematodes 54
Nembutal 118
Neobiotic Aquadrops 106
Neobiotic HC eye drops 68, 113
neomycin 106, 111, 112
neonatal neurological deficits 82
neoplasia, haematuria and 41
Neosulphentrin suspension 106, 111
nipples, sore 30−1
nitrofurantoin 41, 106−7
nutrition 86−96
    dry food 94−6
    during pregnancy 20−1
    principles 86−7
    requirements 95−6
Nuvan Top 6
nystagmus 82
nystatin 62−3, 110, 112

obesity
    ketosis in 22
    pregnancy and 21
occlusion of the penile urethra 42
oestrus 18
    post-partum 19
oil of sassafras 5
Ophthaine 68
Orbenin eye preparation 69
orphans 32−4
osteomyelitis 67
osteoporosis 64
otitis media 73
overcrowding
    mange and 5
    respiratory infections and 46
overheating
    'broken back' and 7

mange and 5
skin problems and 1
oxytocin 117
  agalactica and 31
  dystocia and 26−7
  miscarriage and 23

Panalog
  cream 13, 77, 110, 112
  ophthalmic eye ointment 68,
    77, 113
paralysis 63
Paraspidodera uncinata 54
parturition 25
  complications after 29−32
  complications at 25−9
  skin lesions immediately after 7−8
Pasturella spp. 47, 74, 79
Pasturella multocida 11, 30, 67
penicillin 98
penile urethra, occlusion of 42
pentobarbitone 100−1
Pevidine 62, 77, 97
piperazine 54, 115
plants
  poisonous 91−2
  wild 91−4, 95
pneumonia 2, 46−8
pododermatitis 62−3, 84
poisonous plants 91−2
polydactyly 61
polydipsia, symptoms 40
polyphagia 82
polyuria, symptoms 40−1
post-natal sores 7, 32
post-partum haemorrhage 28
post-partum oestrus 19
povidone-iodine 77, 119−20
praziquantel 55, 116
pregnancy 19−34, 119
  alopecia after 9
  alopecia during 8
  complications during 21−5
  diagnosis 19−20
  exercise during 84
  griseofulvin and 2, 110
  heatstroke and 86
  hormonal maintenance 24−5
  lung abscesses in 47
  mange in 3, 4, 5
  nutritional considerations 20−1
  resorption 22−3

respiratory infections and 46
skin problems in 1
vitamin C and 66, 86
pregnancy toxaemia 21−2, 84, 94,
  109, 116, 117
premature births 24
preputial dermatitis 35
preputial infections 35
preputial prolapse 35
pressure points 62
primidone 4, 82, 118
Probios 108
probiotics 103, 108−9
progesterone 24
propylene glycol 21, 111
protein deficiency 7
Proteus spp. 42
protozoa 54
Pseudomonas aeruginosa 11, 30, 42,
  47
pseudopregnancy, diagnosis 20
pseudotuberculosis 11, 52−3
ptyalism 77

Quellada 4, 115
quickening 19

rabbit food 94
  vitamin C content 1, 87,96
râles 46
rat mange 3
rectum, impaction of 51
red droppings 59
red eye 72
Redoxon 119
rejection of the young 29−30
relaxin 25
renal failure
  acute 43
  chronic 44
  fits and 82
reproductive parameters 17−18
reproductive physiology 17−19
reproductive system 15−38
  anatomy 15−16
reproductive tract 15−16
resorption 22−3
respiratory disorders, symptoms of
  45−6
respiratory infections 46−8
respiratory system 45−8
rhinitis 122

rickets 65
ringworm 1–2, 8, 121
Rompun 100
running lice 5
ruttling 46
  non-infectious 48

Saffan 100
salicylic acid 111
saline solution 11, 12, 35, 61, 73, 93,
    120
  normal 109
salmonella 121–2
Salmonella spp. 24, 52, 121–2
Salmonella enteriditis 51
Salmonella typhimurium 51
Savlon, lip scabs and 7, 78, 120
scabies 4, 114
scent gland 12–13
scours 51
scurvy 9–10, 65–6, 88
sebaceous cyst 11
seborrhoea 2, 8
Seleen, 113
Self-mutilation 4, 7, 99, 100
sellnick 3
septicaemia 51, 82
sexing 17
Shepherd's purse 92, 93
Sherley's Lactol 33
showing, skin problems and 1
Sialitis 78
skin 1–14
  complaints during pregnancy 32
  lesions immediately after
      parturition 7–8
slobbers 77
sneezing 45
snuffles 46
solar dermatitis 73
sow thistle 93
spinach 91
Staphylococcus aureus 11, 30, 62, 67
static lice 5
steroids 100
  cerebellar disease and 83
  diarrhoea and 60
  eye preparation 113
  heatstroke and 86
  mange and 4
  pregnancy toxaemia and 22, 116
stillbirths 25–6

Streptococcus spp. 11, 30, 66, 74
Streptococcus monoiliformis 67, 79
Streptococcus pneumoniae 24, 47, 48
Streptococcus zooepidemicus 47, 78, 105
streptomycin 104
'Stress' 10
stress
  Bordetella outbreaks and 48
  milk flow and 31
sulphamethazine 107, 116
  and coccidiosis 55
  diarrhoea and 58
  haematuria and 41
  non-infectious ruttling and 48
  pneumonia and 47
sulphonamides 111
superfetation 20
surgery
  convalescence 101–2
  post-operative care 101
  preparation for 97
swede 91

Taenia crassicollis 55
Tarlite 8, 9, 118
teeth 74–6
  anatomy 74
  broken 75
  congenital absence 74–75
  weak 75–6
temperature
  high, abortion and 24
  infertility and 85
Tetmosol 4, 114–115
tetracyclines 104–107
thiabendazole, nematodes and 54
Thiostrepton 112
thistle, milk or sow 93
thymus 80
Tinaderm-M cream 110
  pododermatitis and 62–3
  ringworm and 2
toe-nails, overgrown 61
Tolnaftate, 110
  pododermatitis and 63
  ringworm and 2
tooth root abscesses 76
topical preparations 111–2
Torgyl 106, 115
torticollis 46, 74, 79, 82–3
trauma, paralysis and 63
triamcinolone acetonide 112

Tribrissen 41, 107, 108
Trichomonas spp. 54, 115
Trichophyton mentagrophytes 1, 121
tricofolliculomas 13
Trimenopen jenningsi 6
Trixacarus caviae 3, 4, 82, 121
tylosin 98

ulceration, corneal 68, 69, 113
urinary system 39–44
    anatomy 39–40
    physiology 40
urinary tract disorders 40–1
urine-scalding 10–11, 41
urolithiasis 42–3
uterine prolapse 27

vaginal discharge 37–8
vaginal prolapse 28
Valium 118
Vaseline
    corns, pressure points and 62
    impaction of the rectum and 51
    polyuria and 41
    urine-scalding and 11
ventilation, poor, mange and 5
Vetalar 100
vetches 93
Vetrumex 109
    diarrhoea and 58, 60
    pneumonia and 47
Vetsovate 112
    'broken back' and 6
    polyuria and 41
    urine-scalding and 11
Vick vapour rub 34, 47, 81
viral paralysis 63
vitamin B 105
    alopecia and 8
    impaction of the rectum and 51
vitamin B$_{12}$ 119
    miscarriage and 23
    pregnancy toxaemia and 22
vitamin C 119
    in convalescence 101
    deficiency

respiratory infections and 46
    scurvy and 9–10, 66, 88
    skin problems and 1
    wasting disease and 75–6
    diarrhoea and 57
    in pregnancy 20–1
    in rabbit food 96
    requirement 86–7
    wasting disease and 89–90
vitamin D
    deficiency
        rickets and 65
        weak teeth and 75
    osteoporosis and 64
    in rabbit food 96
vitamin E (alpha-tocopherol)
    deficiency 88
    infertility and 36, 89
    muscular dystrophy and 65
vitamin K deficiency 90
    epistaxis and 45
    post-partum haemorrhage and 28
vitamin preparations 118–19
Vitapet
    liver disease and 9
    osteoporosis and 64
    post-natal sores and 7

wasting disease 75–6, 89–90
watercress 91
weaning, hair-loss at 10
Welpi 33
wounds 119, 120
    to the ear 72–3
wry neck 79

yarrow 93, 95
Yersinia 122
Yersinia pseudotuberculosis 52–3
yoghurt, live natural 58, 108
young
    mutilation of 28
    rejection of 29–30
    resorption 22–3

zinc cream 11, 41